三字经小儿推拿

（汉英对照）

Three-Character-Scripture School Pediatric Massage

(Chinese-English)

编著　葛湄菲
Compiled by　Ge Meifei

翻译　单宝枝　郭晓琳
Translated by　Shan Baozhi　Guo Xiaolin

U0308569

中国中医药出版社
·北京·
China Press of Traditional Chinese Medicine
·Beijing·

图书在版编目（CIP）数据

三字经小儿推拿：汉英对照／葛湄菲 编著；单宝枝，
郭晓琳 翻译. — 北京：中国中医药出版社，2016.9
ISBN 978-7-5132-3455-9

Ⅰ.①三… Ⅱ.①葛…②单…③郭… Ⅲ.①小儿疾病－推
拿－汉、英 Ⅳ.① R244.1

中国版本图书馆CIP数据核字（2016）第119907号

中国中医药出版社出版

北京市朝阳区北三环东路28号易亨大厦16层

邮政编码　100013

传真　010 64405750

北京瑞禾彩色印刷有限公司印刷

各地新华书店经销

*

开本 880×1230　1/32　印张 5.5　字数 156千字

2016年9月第1版　2016年9月第1次印刷

书号　ISBN 978-7-5132-3455-9

*

定价 38.00元

网址　www.cptcm.com

前◉言

由于人类疾病谱的变化和健康概念的更新，人们的思维方式、价值观念乃至消费心理、消费行为也发生了变化，使人们对健康水平和生存质量提出了更高的要求，因而目前采用天然药物和自然疗法替代部分化学药品，已成为国际医药发展的普遍动向和趋势。崇尚自然、返璞归真的新型消费，对绿色医疗的需求和期望日益增长。小儿推拿正是迎合了人们对抗生素的担忧和渴望回归自然的心理，越来越受到人们的关注。

三字经流派推拿创建于1877年，其时正值推拿繁荣时期，创始人徐谦光以三个字为一句话，编著《推拿三字经》，由此而得名。学术流派本身就是颇具特色的学术发展过程中的产物，是建立在主流学术基础之上的重要的分支或派别，这种与主流的不同，其实质就是创新，就是发展。三字经流派推拿历经100多年的发展，依然被应用于中医儿科界，是近代小儿推拿疗法中具有代表性的一个流派，在国内外广泛流传，此乃因为它具有自身的特点，主要表现为善用独穴、五脏辨证五行取穴、取穴少而每穴操作时间长、有便于掌握与操作的特定穴、疗效确切重复性强、创造推某穴代替某方剂的独特风格。

绿色消费是人们在对生存环境的担忧、对人们行为反思的基础上提出的，而绿色医疗理念是人们随着生活水平的提高、健康概念的更新和对抗生素的担忧，逐步形成的一种新型医疗消费理念。因此，越来越多的家长为了孩子的健康和将来，会考虑采用没有毒副作用的天然药物和自然疗法，小儿推拿就成为重要的选择之一，这为绿色医疗在儿科应用起到了积极的推动作用。

　　山东省青岛市中医医院儿科自 1955 年建科以来一直沿用三字经流派推拿，使之成为小儿推拿的一大特点，该科室成为山东省中医药重点专科，三字经流派推拿注册了图样商标，三字经流派推拿疗法被列入山东省非物质文化遗产名录。随着来该科室进修、学习人员增多，已出版的《汉英对照三字经流派小儿推拿》再度脱销，为此，笔者结合近年带教的体会，修改了部分内容，使其更贴近于临床，让读者更容易理解，希望三字经流派推拿这一宝贵的非物质文化遗产能更好地服务于广大儿童。

葛湄菲

2016 年 6 月于中国山东青岛

Foreword

As human spectrum of disease is varying and the concept of health is renewing, the way of thinking, the concept of value and even the psychology and behavior of consumers have also changed and higher requirements for health standard and life quality are put forward by people. Some chemical medicines have been substituted by natural medicines and treatments and this has become common trend in the international medicine field. This fresh consumption idea of advocating nature leads to a growing demand and expectation for natural medicine and treatment. Pediatric massage has attracted more and more attention because it meets the needs of people who are unwilling to take antibiotics and eager for going back to nature.

Three-character-scripture School Massage was established in 1877 when massage was just in the boom period. Its founder, *Xu Qianguang*, wrote a book *Three-character Scripture of Massage* with the verses of three Chinese characters becoming a sentence and therefore this school massage was named"Three-character-scripture School Massage". Academic schools are the products in the process of academic development and are important branches based on the mainstream academy. The difference between the branch and mainstream academy is actually innovation and development. Because of its own characteristics, Three-character-scripture School Massage has been developing for more than 100 years, is still used in the TCM pediatrics field, is a representative school in pediatric massage therapy and widespread extensively at home and abroad. Its characteristics are mainly marked by using single point, selecting point based on five elements and five *zang*-organs syndrome differentiation, using fewer points, longer duration of manipulation, easily grasping and manipulating specific points, good efficacy and repeatability, and massaging some point instead of taking some decoction.

Green consumption is put forward based on people's anxiety about the living environment and rethink of their own behaviors, whereas the concept of green medicine and treatments is a gradually developed new concept of medical consumption on the basis of people's high living standard, renewal of the concept of health and anxiety about antibiotics. For the sake of children's health and future, more and more parents are willing to take natural medicines and treatments without toxin and side effects and therefore pediatric massage becomes one of the important choices and plays an active role in the application of the green treatments in children's diseases.

Since the establishment of Pediatric Department of Traditional Chinese Medicine Hospital of *Qingdao* City, *Shandong* province in 1955, Three-character-scripture School Massage has been applying in the department and it has become one major trait of pediatric massage. The department has been approved as one of *Shandong* Provincial Key Characteristic Faculties of Traditional Chinese Medicine. The logo of Three-character-scripture School Massage has been registered. Three-character-scripture School Massage has been included in Intangible Cultural Heritage of *Shandong* Province. With the increase of refresher physicians and visitors, previously published *Chinese-English Edition of Three-Character-Scripture School Pediatric Massage* sold out again and therefore we revise it according to my teaching experience in recent years to make the new edition closer to the clinical practice, and easily understood by readers. I hope the massage serve children better.

Ge Meifei

June 2016, in *Qingdao, Shandong*, China

目⊙录

3

Table of Contents

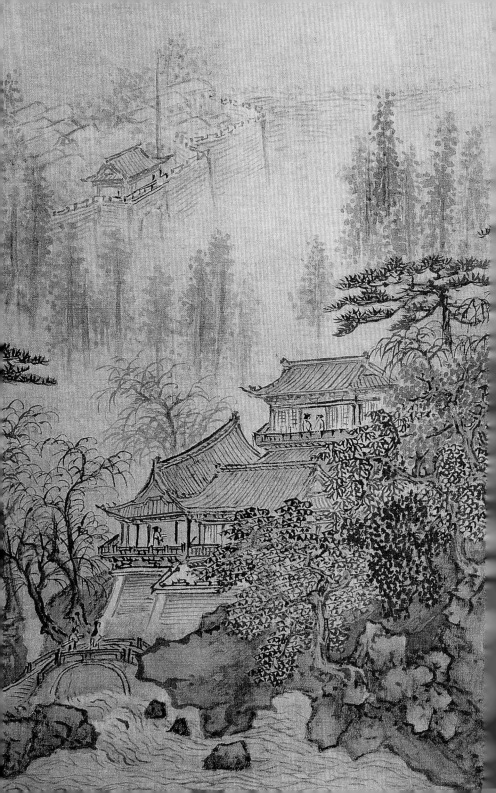

　　中国推拿已有数千年的历史，从远古时代起，按摩术就是我国人民防治疾病的方法之一，特别是隋唐时期，随着医学的迅速发展，按摩疗法发挥了重要作用，成为独立学科。《小儿按摩经》（1601年）的问世，创立了小儿推拿的理论体系，标志着小儿推拿开始了发展的新纪元。后世医家在《小儿按摩经》的基础上不断进行补充，包括穴位、手法、操作方法，加之儿科工作者对小儿的生理病理认识的不断进步，促进了小儿推拿理论及临床实际操作的发展，使小儿推拿的学术思想不断进步以致成熟。而在此发展过程中，由于地域特点引起的人体生理病理的不同，不同医家对此又产生了不同的理解，逐渐发展成为小儿推拿的不同流派，这些不同流派的各家认识，丰富了小儿推拿理论体系，并促进和推动了小儿推拿的理论和临床发展。

一、三字经流派推拿的起源

　　三字经流派推拿自1877年创建后一直在民间盛行，近60年来开始活跃在中医儿科界，近10年，有关创始人的生平与三字经流派推拿的发展的陆续报道，对继承与发展三字经流派推拿起到了积极的推动作用。

　　创始人徐宗礼，字谦光，号秩堂，登郡宁邑人（现山东省牟平宁海镇）。大约生于1820年，卒于何年不详，但光绪七年（1881年）近花甲之年写完家谱。据家谱记载：18岁至京，永兴贸易；道光二十二年（1842年）23岁回家娶亲，仍回京都；道光二十七年（1847年）回家至烟台，开设东文成贸易；虽为商贾，但爱好广泛；经商之旅，亦即学医与悬壶济世之途；博闻而强记，且每有心得则笔耕不缀的习惯为他以后的事业奠定了坚实的基础。

　　同治五年（1866年）因家事而弃商从医，并开始著书，同治十三年（1874年）十二月二十一日，年至半百，历经5年完成《徐氏锦囊》一书。因考虑子孙无能，在书后特注

Massage has a history of several thousand years to prevent and treat diseases in China. In *Sui* and *Tang* dynasties, with the rapid development of TCM, massage treatment played an important role, and became an independent discipline. *Pediatric Massage Classic* was written in 1601, which marked a new era in the development of pediatric massage, and the theoretical system of pediatric massage was founded. The doctors of later generations updated the system in points, manipulations, method of operation constantly on the basis of the book mentioned above and the pediatricians understood the physiological and pathological characteristics of children further clearly, which promoted the development of the theory and clinical operations of pediatric massage and therefore the academic thought of pediatric massage improved and matured constantly. During the process of development, different doctors had different understanding of different physiological and pathological characteristics caused by different geographical features, different schools of pediatric massage were gradually founded. Such different understanding of different schools enriched the theoretical system of the pediatric massage and played a positive role in the development of the theory and clinic of pediatric massage.

1　Origin of Three-character-scripture School Massage

Three-character-scripture School Massage was established in 1877, with its popularity among the folk. It became active in the TCM field of pediatrics about 60 years ago. Recently, many books about the development of Three-character-scripture School Massage and the life of initiator have been reported, which plays an active role in the inheritance and development of the Three-character-scripture School Massage.

The initiator, *Xu Zongli*, from *Ninghai* town, *Mouping* district, *Shandong* province, was born in 1820. He accomplished his Family Tree Manual in 1881. According to the Family Tree Manual, after he got married at the age of 23, he went to Peking, the capital city. In 1847, he established East *Wencheng* Trade in *Yantai* city of *Shandong* province. Though a businessman, he had a wide range of interest, especially in the field of TCM. Moreover, his open horizon, thirst for knowledge and a good habit of writing down his sense perception laid a solid foundation for his later success.

3

"徐氏锦囊万两不售，以为传家之至宝也"。此书至今保存在徐氏家族中。

《推拿三字经》著成于1877年。徐谦光因母病服药即吐，在此情况下，运用了小儿推拿手法而获效，在不断的临证实践中逐步形成了自己的一套推拿疗法，和一般的推拿多有不同，只用推手的方法，通治大人和小儿诸病。作者为了使此书广为流传，而未在家中保存。《推拿三字经》手抄本现存于山东中医药大学图书馆。

此书虽未出版，但在民间流行很广，其孙子徐克善继承祖业，在山东烟台地区成为小儿推拿名医，但其后未有传人。将三字经流派推拿发扬光大当数山东省青岛市中医医院李德修先生。

二、三字经流派推拿的传承

李德修（1893—1972年），又名慎之，山东威海市北竹岛村人。幼时家贫辍学，在渔船上学徒，以打工为生，17岁染疾，暴致耳聋，幸遇威海清泉学校校长戚经含，怜其疾苦，遂赠清代徐谦光著的《推拿三字经》一书，并悉心指教，经8年学习，方独立应诊。1920年来青岛，在鸿祥钱庄设诊所，以推拿疗疾，颇具声望。1929年自设诊所，求治者盈门。1955年应聘到山东省青岛市中医医院工作，任小儿科负责人。

建院初期，医院领导安排护士孙爱兰、刘瑞英跟随李德修学习推拿技术，虽无明确的师承关系，但临床诊治和推拿手法均在李德修亲自指导下完成，可谓是李德修的传人，1962年、1963年先后收本院医师王德芝、王安岗为徒。刘瑞英是在李德修身边工作时间最长的人员，自1955年7月至1990年11月退休，一直在儿科从事小儿推拿工作，一生中没有留下著作，但在三字经流派推拿的传承中，起着承上启下的作用。作者1983年在青岛市中医医院儿科跟随刘瑞英学习小儿推拿，2001年调入该科室任儿科主任。

In 1866, he went back home for something happening in his family. From then on, he took medical work and dedicated his time to write books. He spent 5 years to have *Xu's Wise Counsels* finished on 21st, Dec. 1874, by which time, he was in his fifties. Considering the inability of his offspring, he noted in the end of his book: I take *Xu's Wise Counsels* as a family heirloom, it is priceless, not for sale. Up to now, this book is still kept by *Xu*'s offspring.

Three-character-scripture School Massage was completed in 1877. *Xu* cured his mother with massage on the ground that she vomited while taking medicines. He founded his own massage method during his constant clinical practice, which is quite different from common massage. He massaged on hand only and it was suitable for both children and adults. The manuscript of *Three-character-scripture School Massage* is now kept in the library of *Shandong* University of TCM.

Although the book was not published, its handwritten copies were then widely popular. *Xu Keshan*, *Xu*'s grandson, became a famous pediatric massager in *Yantai*, *Shandong* province, but he had no successor. Afterwards *Li Dexiu*, a doctor of *Qingdao* TCM Hospital, *Shandong* province, carried forward the Three-character-scripture School Massage.

2 Inheritance of Three-character-scripture School Massage

Li Dexiu (1893—1972), also called *Shenzhi*, was born in *Zhudao* village, *Weihai*, *Shandong* province, he was poor and discontinued his studies when he was young. He earned a living on a fishing boat as an apprentice before he got sudden deafness due to a disease at the age of 17. Luckily, *Qi Jinghan*, the headmaster of *Qingquan* School of *Weihai* city, sympathized with his misfortune by teaching him with *Xu Zongli's* Three-character-scripture School Massage and giving him advice heartily. After 8 years of hard study, *Li* was able to treat diseases by himself. In 1920, he went to *Qingdao* and worked in a clinic under *Hongxiang* Private Bank, where he made fame by treating diseases with massage. In 1929, he set up his own clinic with affluent patients. In 1953, he practiced medicine in a dwelling of *Guanhai* Road. In 1955, he was nominated as the Director of the department of pediatrics in *Qingdao* TCM Hospital, *Shandong* province.

三、三字经流派推拿的文献传承

作为中医学术流派，除了以人来承载的形式外，还有以文献来承载的形式。只有传人而没有文献的东西大多只能归入技巧之类，只有文献而没有传人的学术亦无疑是绝学。三字经流派推拿历经 100 多年依然活跃在中医儿科界，就是因为它不仅以人来承载，而且也以文献为承载。

《推拿三字经》：1877 年徐谦光著，未出版，手抄本现存于山东中医药大学图书馆。此书除序言之外，主要为三字一句歌诀。为此被后人称为三字经流派推拿。

《小儿推拿三字经》：1958 年青岛市中医医院油印，内部刊物。此书根据李德修所存手抄本整理而成，与原著基本相同，只是注释较原著多。

《李德修小儿推拿技法》：1984 年王蕴华著，未出版，青岛市中医医院内部刊物。此书真实而客观地记录了李德修的推拿技巧与临床经验，在三字经流派推拿传承中起到重要作用。

At the beginning of the establishment of the TCM hospital, leaders arranged two nurses, *Sun Ailan* and *Liu Ruiying*, to study *Li Dexiu*'s massage technique. Though there was no clear master and apprentice relationship, both of them acquired technique of clinical diagnosis and massage manipulation under the guidance of *Li*. It could be said that they were apprentices of *Li Dexiu*. *Li Dexiu* received *Wang Dezhi*, *Wang Angang*, the doctors of *Qingdao* hospital of TCM, as apprentices in 1962 and in 1963. *Liu Ruiying* has been working with *Li Dexiu* from July 1955 to November 1990. She has been a pediatric massager in Pediatric Clinic, and has no literary work, however, she played the role of a connecting link in the inheritance of Three-character-scripture School Massage. I followed *Liu Ruiying* learning pediatric massage at *Qingdao* TCM hospital in 1983, and became the director of the pediatric department of the hospital in 2001.

3 Heritage Literature of Three-character-scripture School Massage

Inheritance of the schools includes inheritors and heritage literature. Having inheritors without heritage literature is classified as skill while having heritage literature without inheritors is called lost knowledge. Three-character-scripture School Massage is still active in the TCM pediatrics field after more than 100 years of development because it has both inheritors and heritage literature.

Three-character Scripture of Massage was completed by *Xu Zongli* in 1877 and it was not published. Its manuscript is kept in the library of *Shandong* University of TCM now. The book was in the form of verses with three Chinese characters making one sentence except the preface. So the massage is called Three-character-scripture School Massage.

Three-character Scripture of Pediatric Massage was printed as internal data by *Qingdao* TCM hospital in 1958 and it was revised on the basis of *Li Dexiu*'s handwritten copy. It was basically the same as the original while it had just more notes as compared with the original.

Li Dexiu's Techniques of Pediatric Massage written by *Wang Yunhua* in 1984 was printed as internal data. In the book, *Li Dexiu*'s massage techniques and clinical experience were recorded truly and objectively. It played an important role in the inheritance of Three-character-scripture

7

《幼科推拿三字经派求真》：1992年赵鉴秋著，青岛出版社出版。此书重点是小儿常见病推拿治疗、小儿保健推拿、小儿脏腑点穴法，其中，小儿常见病推拿内容约占64%，属于三字经流派推拿。而其书后《推拿三字经》浅释，基本上是1958年青岛市中医医院油印本的注解。

《汉英对照三字经流派小儿推拿》：2008年葛湄菲编著，上海科学技术出版社出版。此书在王蕴华《李德修小儿推拿技法》基础上，结合小儿的生理病理特点，对小儿常见病、多发病逐步进行规范化治疗，采用汉英对照形式，有利于三字经流派推拿走向世界。

四、三字经流派推拿的发展

作者自2001年调入青岛市中医医院儿科，用了近5年的时间，先后到济南、牟平、威海等地进行了实地考察，主要方式为查阅档案馆资料，走访创始人的后人及三字经流派继承人的后人，真实而客观地记录发展史。2008年完成了"三字经流派推拿文献整理研究"课题，该课题系统整理了三字经流派推拿的起源与发展，首次报道了创始人的生平，明确了三字经流派的传承，较完整、准确地整理了《推拿三字经》中的推拿部分；"三字经流派小儿推拿临床技术研究"课题从临床取穴、操作方法及操作时间等多方面，与《推拿学》（高等医药院校教材，俗称五版教材）对比分析，系统总结了三字经流派推拿临床特点；同年出版了《汉英对照三字经流派小儿推拿》专著，完成了三字经流派推拿文献传承工作。

School Massage.

The Essence of Three-character Scripture of Pediatric Massage written by *Zhao Jianqiu* was published by *Qingdao* Publishing House in 1992. The book focused on such contents as massage therapy of common pediatric diseases, pediatric healthcare massage, pediatric *Zang-fu* point-massaging method, in which the content of massage therapy of common pediatric diseases covered about 64 percent. Brief elucidation of *Three-character Scripture of Massage* was attached to the last part of the book.

Chinese-English Edition of Three-character-scripture School Pediatric Massage written by *Ge Meifei* in 2008 was published by *Shanghai* Scientific and Technical Publishers. Based on *Wang Yunhua's Li Dexiu's Techniques of Pediatric Massage* and the children's physiological and pathological features, standardized treatments for common pediatric diseases were recorded in the book. Chinese-English edition of it is helpful for the massage to go globally.

4 Development of Three-character-scripture School Massage

I have worked in *Qingdao* TCM Hospital from 2001 and has spent nearly five years to do field visits in *Jinan*, *Mouping*, *Weihai* and other places, mainly checked out the data of archives, visited the initiator's descendants and the descendants of the inheritors of Three-character-scripture School Pediatric Massage, and recorded the history truly and objectively. A subject named Literature Collection and Study on Three-character-scripture School Massage was completed in 2008. In the subject, the origin and development of Three-character-scripture School Massage was collected systematically, the founder's life was reported for the first time, the inheritance of Three-character-scripture School Massage was made clear, the part of massage of Three-character –scripture School Massage was collected completely and exactly. Another subject named Clinical Techniques Research of Three-character-scripture School Massage involved the contrast and analysis in the aspects of clinical point selection, methods of operation, operating time and so on compared with *Science of Massage* — one of the Higher Education Medical and Pharmaceutical University Textbooks and the systematic summary of the clinical features of Three-character-scripture School Massage. At the

2007 年作者申请注册了三字经流派推拿图样商标，2008 年作为青岛市卫生行业中医特色专科，进入国家中医药管理局"十一五"重点专科协作组，作为"三字经流派推拿治疗小儿泄泻的临床验证"牵头单位，在全国 5 家三级甲等中医院完成了临床验证工作，证明了三字经流派推拿治疗小儿泄泻的临床疗效和安全性，使三字经流派小儿推拿技术在全国各地得以更好地顺利推广。2011 年三字经流派推拿技术成为山东省卫生行业适宜技术推广项目，三字经流派推拿疗法 2012 年、2013 年分别列入市级、省级非物质文化遗产名录，作者被评为市级、省级非物质文化遗产项目"三字经流派推拿疗法"代表性传承人。

五、三字经流派推拿的学术特点

三字经流派推拿历经 100 多年而长盛不衰，就是因为它与其他流派相比具有独创性，主要表现在善用独穴、五脏辨证五行取穴、取穴少而每穴操作时间长、具有便于掌握与操作的特定穴、疗效确切且重复性强、创造推某穴代替某方的独特风格。以原著为准，概述其学术特点。

1. 通治成人与小儿

徐谦光所用的推拿穴位通治成人与小儿，原著从开始就说明他研究推拿的动机，第 1～4 句"徐谦光奉萱堂药无缘推拿恙"，第 15～20 句"大三万小三千婴三百加减良分岁数轻重当"。明确地指出，他的母亲有病，服药即吐，不能用药物治疗，才采用了推拿疗法，他书中的内容亦是成人小儿通治。他将 16～100 岁的称为大人；5～15 岁为小儿；3～5 岁为婴儿；0～3 岁为幼婴，治疗中以手法的轻重与时间的长短为区别，特别是手法方面，成人速而重，小儿速而轻；推的时间，成人长而小儿短。将小儿推拿手法扩充用于成人病，这是与其他小儿推拿著作最大的不同。

same year, *Chinese-English Edition of Three-character-scripture School Pediatric Massage* was published and the literature inheritance work was completed.

The logo of Three-character-scripture School Massage was registered in 2007. The pediatric department of *Qingdao* TCM Hospital was selected as one of the TCM characteristic departments of *Qingdao* health industry and was included as "Eleventh Five-Year-Plan" Key Characteristic Departments Collaborative Group approved by the SATCM (State Administration of Traditional Chinese Medicine of the People's Republic of China) in 2008. As a leading unit, our hospital completed the clinical verifications about Treating Pediatric Diarrhea with Three-character-scripture School Massage in 5 top three hospitals. The clinical efficacy and safety were proved and therefore the technique of Three-character-scripture School Massage was popularized smoothly. The technique of Three-character-scripture School Massage was selected as the suitable project of *Shandong* provincial health industry to be popularized in 2011. Three-character-scripture School Massage was approved as *Qingdao* Intangible Cultural Heritage in 2012 and as *Shandong* Intangible Cultural Heritage in 2013 and I was selected as its representative inheritor of Three-character-scripture School Massage.

5 Academic Features of Three-character-scripture School Massage

Since established in 1877 and developed for more than 100 years, Three-character-scripture School Massage has been widely used due to its originality compared with other schools massage. Its unique styles are using single point, syndrome differentiation and treatment based on five *zang*-organs and five elements, selecting less point, long duration of manipulation, easily grasping specific points, obvious curative effect, good repeatability, and the creation of using some point instead of some formula. The academic features of Three-character-scripture School Massage are outlined based on the original.

5.1 The massage is applicable to both children and adults

The points which *Xu* selected can be used to treat children and adults.

11

2．善用独穴治急症

第25～28句"治急病一穴良大数万立愈恙"，第81～84句"若泻肚推大肠一穴愈来往忙"，第97～100句"若腹痛窝风良数在万立无恙"。徐氏擅长于独穴治病，就是只用一个穴位，多推、久推，以得效为度，特别是急性病，更主张用独穴，事实证明这一疗法是有效的，且是其他推拿流派所不具备的。

3．取穴少而每穴操作时间长

一般推拿疗法是全身取穴，穴位至少也在80个以上，治疗一种病常用到10个穴位以上，而徐氏列举的穴位只有44个，其中有10个穴位一般不用，因此，徐氏常用的穴位不过34个，不到一般推拿疗法采用穴位的一半，在治疗疾病中只用1～2个穴位，至多也不过5个穴位；一般推拿因采用的穴位多，每个穴位只推1～2分钟，最多不过5分钟，总的推拿时间是长的，徐氏采用的穴位极少，而特别主张每个穴推的时间长，总的推拿时间与一般推拿疗法相同（主要指小儿推拿）。如：第173～180句记载："脱肛者肺虚恙补脾土二马良补肾水推大肠来回推久去恙。"对于脱肛者采用补脾经、揉二马、补肾经、清补大肠穴，"久去恙"的久字，即代表每次操作时间长，也提示治疗的疗程长。也不难看出三字经流派推拿手法以推法、揉法最为常用，手法归纳起来，只有推、揉、捣、拿、分合、运6种手法，容易学习和掌握，便于推广和应用。

He had explained his motivation of massage research at the beginning of the original. In No.1-4 and No.15-20 sentences of his book, it was explicitly showed that his mother was sick and she vomited whiling taking medicines, so he treated her with massage. Treating the adults and children was recorded in his book. The persons at 16-100 years of age are defined as adults; at 5-15 years of age, as teenage, at 3-5 years of age, as children; at 0-3 years of age, as infants. Generally, fast and powerful manipulation is for the adults while fast and light one for children. Longer duration is for the adults while shorter duration for children. The biggest difference between Three-character-scripture School Massage and others is that the former is expanded by using its manipulation on adults.

5.2 Being good at treating emergency with single point

In No.25-28 and No.81-84 sentences of the original, it was showed that *Xu* was good at treating diseases with single point, namely only using one point to treat diseases. Generally, the manipulation needed longer duration and did not stop until it worked, especially suitable for emergency. The therapy had been proved to be effective, and different from other schools massage.

5.3 Selecting fewer points and longer duration of manipulation

In other massage, the selection of points is all over the body and at least 80 points can be involved for common application and over 10 points for one disease each time. However, the *Xu*'s massage discussed only 44 points and among them, 10 points were not commonly used and therefore 34 points were normally involved by *Xu* and only 1-2 points or at most 5 points were applied to treat disease each time. In manipulation, more points are usually selected each time and the duration of manipulation on each point is short, only 1-2 minutes, or at most 5 minutes for other schools massage while fewer points are selected each time and the duration of manipulation on each point is long for *Xu*'s massage. For example, in No.173-180 sentences of the original, it was recorded that he used nourishing spleen-meridian point, kneading *erma* point, nourishing kidney-meridian point, and harmonizing large-intestine-meridian point to treat rectocele. The original sentence hinted that the therapy included longer duration of manipulation and longer course of treatment. It was

13

4．流派的特定穴与操作

三字经流派小儿推拿（以下称流派推拿）特定穴的操作位置与《推拿学》五版教材的小儿推拿（以下称教学推拿）有所不同，流派推拿四横纹的位置是第 2～5 指掌指关节横纹，操作时来回推，称推四横纹，相当于教学推拿的小横纹，教学推拿四横纹的位置为掌面示指、中指、无名指、小指第 1 指间关节横纹处。流派推拿胃经穴的位置在第 1 掌骨桡侧缘赤白肉际处，教学推拿胃经的位置是在拇指掌面近掌端第 1 节。流派推拿脾经的位置是拇指桡侧缘赤白肉际处，肝经穴、心经穴、肺经穴、肾经穴的位置分别在示指、中指、无名指、小指掌面，从指尖到指根，教学推拿脾经穴、肝经穴、心经穴、肺经穴、肾经穴的位置分别在拇指、示指、中指、无名指、小指末节罗纹面。

特定穴在操作上也有很大的不同。流派推拿中的脾经穴、肝经穴、心经穴、肺经穴、肾经穴均为线型穴位，从指尖推向指根为补（向心为补），从指根推向指尖为清（离心为清）；教学推拿脾经穴、肝经穴、心经穴、肺经穴旋推为补，向指根方向直推为清（向心为清）；肾经穴由指根向指尖方向直推为补（离心为补），由指尖向指根方向直推为清（向心为清）。

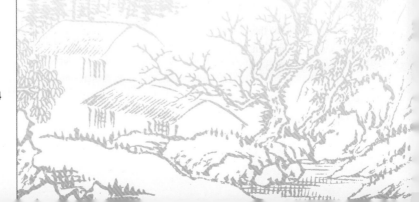

also showed that there are only six kinds of commonly used manipulations including pushing, kneading, pounding, grasping, parting-pushing & meeting pushing, and arc-pushing and among them, pushing and kneading are the most commonly used ones in Three-character-scripture School Massage. It is easy to learn and grasp, promote and apply.

5.4 Specific points and manipulation

The manipulation location of specific points is different between Three-character-scripture School Massage (abbreviation: school massage) and *Science of Massage* — one of the Higher Education Medical and Pharmaceutical University Textbooks (abbreviation: teaching massage). For example, in school massage, the four-transverse-crease point is a linear point with the whole line of the transverse crease of the finger root of the index, middle, third and little fingers. In manipulation, push it to and fro. It is equivalent to little-transverse-crease point of teaching massage. The four-transverse-crease point of teaching massage is a linear point with the whole line of the transverse crease of the first interphalangeal joint stripes of the index, middle, third and little fingers. The stomach-meridian point of school massage is a linear point in the dorso-ventral boundary of the lateral side of the big thenar from transverse crease of the wrist to the root of the thumb while is the thenar muscles in teaching massage. The spleen-meridian point of school massage is a linear point along the lateral side of the thumb, from its tip to root while is in fingerprint surfaces of thumb in teaching massage. The liver-meridian point, heart-meridian point, lung-meridian point and kidney-meridian point of school massage are linear points along the ventral side of the index, middle, third and little fingers from its tip to root while are in fingerprint surfaces of the middle finger distal of the index, middle, third and little fingers in teaching massage.

There are also a lot of different operations on specific points. The spleen-meridian point, the liver-meridian point, the lung-meridian point, and the kidney-meridian point of school massage are linear points, pushing from its root to tip (centrifugal pushing) usually has the function of clearing while pushing from its tip to root (centripetal pushing) is nourishing. Arc-pushing the spleen-meridian point, the liver-meridian point, the heart-meridian point and the lung-meridian point of teaching

15

5．偏重望诊及五脏辨证

中医诊法，离不开望闻问切四诊。然而小儿口不能言，脉无所察，唯形色以为凭，故历代儿科医家均将望诊列为四诊之首。徐氏在书中对切脉略微一提，而在望诊方面讨论独详，这样，对儿科诊断方面就有了较大的帮助，因望诊而联系到五脏，就强调了五脏辨证。"大察脉理宜详浮沉者表里恙迟数者冷热伤寒内外推无恙虚与实仔细详字廿七脉诀讲明四字治诸恙小婴儿看印堂五色纹细心详"。（35～52句）徐氏诊查方法是用水洗净小儿印堂，然后观察色泽。红色热在心肺，紫则热甚，青则为肝有风热，黑则为风寒入骨，白色为肺有痰，黄色为病在脾。五色结合五脏，大体就可以找出病在何脏，运用八纲辨证确定治则。

6．治疗取穴以五行生克为原则

徐氏认为，学习推拿法，首须掌握五行生克原则。"虚补母实泻子曰五行生克当生我母我生子穴不误治无恙"。（329～336句）肾水生肝木，肝木生心火，心火生脾土，脾土生肺金，肺金生肾水，此为五行配五脏相生的规律；五行相克，则为水克火，火克金，金克木，木克土，土克水。生我者为母，我生者为子，其关系极为密切，治疗理法亦寓于其中，如肾水生肝木，肾水亏不能涵木，肝亦必虚，龙雷之火必然上沸；肝木生心火，木不能生火则心血亏而血亦必寒。虚则补其母，如肝虚可以补肾；实则泻其子，肝热者可清泻心火，心经穴不宜外推，用天河水穴即可。掌握此理，选穴不误，自能得效。

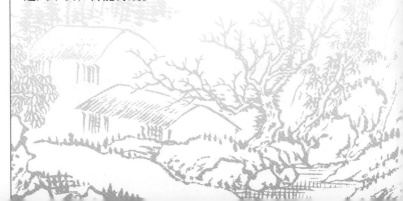

massage is nourishing while pushing from its tip to root (centripetal pushing) is clearing. Kidney-meridian point is an exception, pushing from its root to tip (centrifugal pushing) is nourishing while pushing from its tip to root (centripetal pushing) has the function of clearing.

5.5 Emphasis on inspection and syndrome differentiation based on five *zang*-organs

Diagnostic methods in TCM include inspection, listening and smelling, inquiry and pulse-taking. But an infant cannot speak, his/her pulse cannot be examined, it is diagnosed according to looking only. So inspection is listed as the first of four diagnostic methods by pediatricians of past dynasties. *Xu* also paid attention to inspection and syndrome differentiation based on five *zang*-organs. In No. 35-52 sentences of the original, *Xu's* method of inspection lies in washing the infant's *yintang* and then observing the color. Red indicates heat in the heart and lung, purple means heavy heat, green shows heat and wind in the liver, black indicates cold and wind into bones, white means phlegm in the lung, yellow means sickness in the spleen. By way of five colors combining five *zang*-organs, he could find where the sickness was, determined the treating principles according to eight-principle syndrome differentiation.

5.6 Selecting point according to the principles of the relations of generation and restriction in five elements

Xu believed that massage should be learned after grasping the principles of the relations of generation and restriction in five elements. In No.329-336 sentences of the original, the principles of five elements matching generation of five *zang*-organs were that the kidney water generated liver wood, liver wood generated heart fire, heart fire generated spleen earth, spleen earth generated lung gold, lung gold generated kidney water, while the principles of five elements matching restriction of five *zang*-organs were that water restricted fire, fire restricted gold, gold restricted wood, wood restricted earth, earth restricted water. Generating is mother, being generated is son, which the relation is very close and resided in the principle and rule of the treatment. For example, the kidney water generated liver wood, deficiency of kidney water could not generate liver wood, leading to deficiency of liver wood, *longlei* fire would ascend.

17

7．独创推某穴代替某方剂

徐氏主张用独穴治病，独创了根据治疗的需要，某种病专推某一个穴，以多推来取效的方法，并制定了推拿26个穴位代替26种方剂的方案，形成了三字经流派推拿的独特风格，其特点以推某穴代某方剂，与《幼科铁镜》中以推某穴代某药不同。如："分阴阳为水火两治汤；推三关为参附汤；退六腑为清凉散；天河水为安心丹；运八卦调中益气汤……"

三字经流派小儿推拿临床疗效高，手法简单易学，重复性强，越来越受到重视，使其在全国乃至世界产生了广泛的影响。加强三字经流派小儿推拿临床研究与推广，让中医学的这一宝贵遗产更好地服务于广大儿童，是我们的责任。

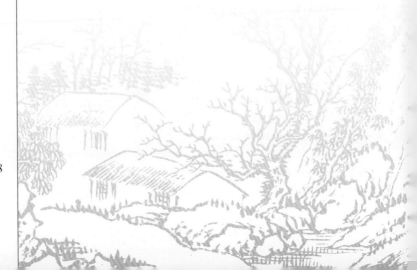

The liver wood generated heart fire, if wood could not generate fire, heart blood would be deficient and the blood would be cold. Because deficiency needed nourishing its mother-organ, such as, nourishing liver through nourishing kidney; excess needed clearing its son-organ, such as clearing liver fire through clearing heart fire, but heart-meridian point cannot be touched directly, clearing heaven-river-water point can be selected instead. Grasp the principles, select right points, and therefore the therapy can do work.

5.7 Massaging some point instead of some formula created by Xu

Xu advocated using single point to treat disease, created the original method of using one point and longer duration of manipulation each time according to the need to treat some disease, and applied 26 points instead of 26 formulae respectively. It is the unique style of Three-character-scripture School Massage, which is different from the method of massaging some point instead of some herb in the *You Ke Tie Jing*. For example, in Three-character-scripture School Massage, "Parting-*yin-yang* point is equivalent to *Shui Huo Liang Zhi* Decoction, pushing *sanguan* point is equivalent to *Shen Fu* Decoction, clearing manipulation on six-*fu* point is equivalent to *Liang Ge* Powder, clearing manipulation on heaven-river-water point is equivalent to *An Xin* Pills, arc-pushing *bagua* point is equivalent to *Tiao Zhong Yi Qi* Decoction and so on."

Three-character-scripture School Pediatric Massage attracts more and more attention and impacts widely in China even in the world on the ground that it is of highly curative effect, easily grasping, and good repeatability. It is our duty to enhance clinical research and promotion of the massage, let the precious heritage of TCM serve our children better.

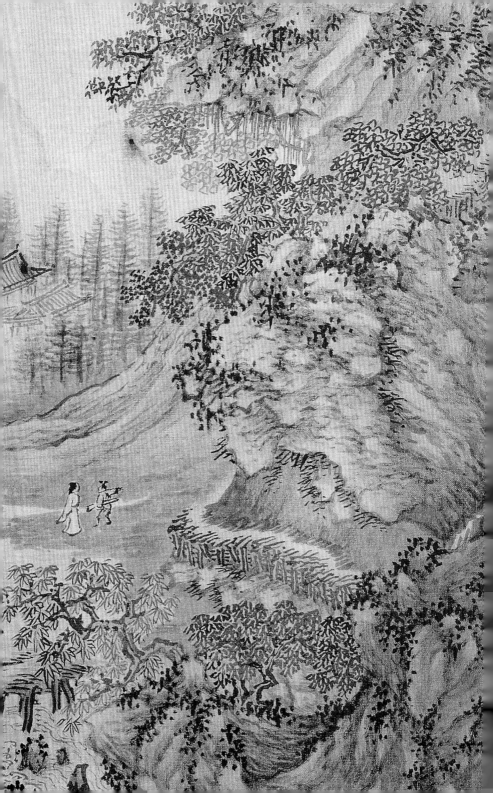

Chapter 2
Basic Theory of the Pediatric Massage

第二章
小儿推拿基本理论

小儿推拿的作用原理是医生根据病情，以不同的、轻柔的推拿手法作用于人体体表的特定部位从而调节机体的生理病理状况，达到治疗和保健的目的。小儿推拿手法是良性的、有序的和具有双向调节性的物理刺激，易被小儿内脏或形体感知，从而产生功效。小儿推拿历经几千年的发展，在历代医家的反复推敲检验下，去伪存真，各种手法切实可靠而行之有效，并形成了完整的体系，隶属于中医学范畴，所以，小儿推拿的作用原理可以从中医学的角度去认识探讨。

一、小儿推拿的作用原理

阴阳五行、营卫气血和经络学说，是推拿疗法的理论基础。凡脏腑、骨肉、经络以至于皮毛，莫不由气血滋养，而经络是气血循环的路径，经络之气又能促进气血的运行。小儿推拿是应用各种手法作用在体表特定穴位上，通过经络"行气血，通阴阳"的作用，达到和脏腑、畅气机的治疗疾病的目的。

中医学认为，阴阳可以概括人体内部一切矛盾斗争和变化，疾病就是阴阳失调的结果，故而治疗疾病，应当调整阴阳，使之趋于平衡，《黄帝内经》说"阴平阳秘，精神乃治"亦即此意。推拿是通过以下几方面的作用原理达到调整阴阳的目的。

1. 推拿调整阴阳

人体腧穴可以分阳穴与阴穴。阳穴位于阳分，如手背、前臂桡侧、背部、下肢外侧等；阴穴位于阴分，如手掌、前臂尺侧、腹部、下肢内侧。一般而言，阳病治阴，阴病治阳。

How does the pediatric massage work? Actually, to achieve treatment and healthcare aims, a manipulator applies different and gentle *tuina* (massage) manipulations to the specific points on the surface of human body to adjust the physiological and pathological conditions of organism according to child's condition. The pediatric massage manipulation is a sort of healthy, orderly physical stimulation with bidirectional adjusting effect, and is easily perceptible by internal organs or body of children and therefore it works. With the development of it, the pediatric massage has been deliberated, tested and revised repeatedly by many doctors in generations for thousands of years. A variety of manipulations has been made reliable and effective and has formed a complete system which pertains to the category of traditional Chinese medicine (TCM). Its action principle could be understood and discussed from a TCM viewpoint.

1 Action Principle of the Pediatric Massage

The theoretical basis of the massage covers *yin-yang* and five elements theory, *ying, wei, qi, xue* (nutrient-defense-*qi*-blood) theory, and channel and collateral theory. *Qi* and blood nourish *zang-fu organs*, bone & flesh, meridian and skin-hair. Channel and collaterals are the paths of *qi* and blood circulation, and the *qi* of channel and collaterals can promote *qi* and blood to run. A pediatric massage manipulator applies a variety of manipulations to the specific points on the surface of child's body to make *zang-fu organs* be in harmony and *qi* movement smooth by the action of the channel and collaterals on *qi*-blood and *yin-yang*.

TCM holds that all of the contradictions, struggles and changes in the body can be summarized by *yin-yang*. Diseases result in *yin-yang* disorder. So treatment of disease should adjust *yin-yang* to balance. It is the meaning of "only when *yin* is at peace and *yang* is compact can essence-spirit be normal." in *Huangdi Neijing*. The action principle of the pediatric massage is discussed in detail as follows:

1.1 Adjusting *yin* and *yang*

Human points include *yang* points and *yin* points. *Yang* points lie in *yang* aspect, such as opisthenar, radial forearm, back, the lateral of the lower limbs and so on; *Yin* points lie in *yin* aspect, such as palm, ulnar

23

　　小儿推拿操作，根据阴阳的相互关系创立了调整阴阳的方法。如分阴阳、合阴阳之法，如《推拿秘书》所言："推此不特能和气血，凡一切臌胀、泄泻，如五脏六腑有虚，或大小便不通，或惊风痰喘等疾，皆可治之。至于乍寒乍热，尤为对症。热多，则分阳从重，寒多，则分阴从重。"认为分阴阳及合阴阳可以调理脏腑、阴阳、气血；如三关与六腑穴，一热甚一寒甚，在应用时可以按比例配合应用，可以达到调整寒热阴阳的作用；在具体穴位的操作上有顺运与逆运法，如内八卦穴，顺运可以开胸膈、除胀满，逆运八卦可以降气平喘。

2. 推拿顺应升降

　　推拿可以调整气机，顺应气机升降，一般而言，肝主升，肺主降，脾居中焦，主斡旋气机，升清降浊，以助肝升肺降。而病理状态下，肺当降不降则为咳嗽气喘，肝当升不升则为头晕目眩，而脾虚升清降浊失职，升清不及则有飧泻，降浊不及则为膜胀。因此治疗之时，应当顺应这种升降的趋势使用手法。三字经流派小儿推拿的穴位，以线状穴位为主，其升降也是有规律可循的。如：线性穴位向上（向心）推是升，向下（离心）推是降，脾经向上（向心）推为补，胃经向下（离心）推为清，三关向上（向心）推有升阳益气的作用，六腑向下（离心）推有清热祛邪的作用。

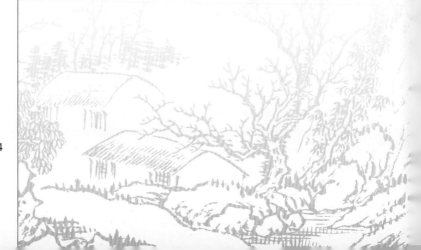

forearm, abdomen and the inside of the lower limbs. Generally, treat *yin* for the *yang* disease, treat *yang* for the *yin* disease.

The method of adjusting the *yin-yang* was founded according to the mutual relationship of *yin* and yang in the manipulation of pediatric massage, such as parting-*yin-yang* and meeting-*yin-yang*. "Massage can be applied to the treatment of abdominal distension, diarrhea, deficiency syndrome in five *zang*-organs and six *fu*-organs, constipation, urine retention, infantile convulsions and phlegm panting, especially alternative chilliness and fever. More heat, more parting-*yang*; More cold, more parting-*yin*." in *Massage Esoteric*, an ancient massage book. It holds that parting-*yin-yang* and meeting-*yin-yang* have the functions of adjusting *zang-fu*, *yin-yang*, and *qi-xue*; such as *Sanguan* point (warm point) and six-*fu* point (cold point) are applied together proportionally to regulate cold-heat and *yin-yang*. There are clockwise arc-pushing and anticlockwise arc-pushing manipulations used in specific points. For example, clockwise arc-pushing *bagua* point is of the action of eliminating flatulence in the chest and anticlockwise arc-pushing *bagua* point descending *qi* and relieving dyspnea.

1.2 Conforming to the ascending and descending of *qi* movement

Massage can be applied to regulate *qi* movement, and conform to the ascending and descending of *qi* movement. Generally, the liver governs to ascend, the lung to descend; the spleen lying in the middle-*jiao* mediates *qi* movement, and ascend lucidity and descend turbidity to help the liver to ascend and the lung to descend. However, under the pathological conditions, the lung fails to descend, cough and dyspnea occur, the liver fails to ascend, dizziness. If the spleen is insufficient and fails to ascend lucidity and descend turbidity, diarrhea with undigested food will develop caused by lucidity-underascending of the spleen, abdominal distension caused by turbidity-underdescending of the speen. So the massage manipulation should be selected to follow the trend of ascending or descending. The points of three-character-scripture school pediatric massage are mainly linear points, there are rules to comply with regarding their ascending and descending. For example, pushing down (centrifugal direction) on the linear points pertains to descending while pushing up (centripetal direction) pertains to ascending. Pushing up (centripetal

25

3．推拿补虚泻实

推拿可以补虚泻实。对于正气不足之虚证，选用有补益作用的穴位可以增强脏腑功能，提高其兴奋性，称为补法，如脾虚泄泻，重用补脾经，可以恢复脾胃运化升清的功能；对于邪气有余之实证，选用有祛邪作用的穴位可以抑制脏腑功能，降低其兴奋性，称为泻法，如湿热泄泻，可以重用清大肠经，以祛除湿热之邪，恢复正常大便规律。

另外，根据操作手法的力度、时间以及手法频率、操作方向可分为轻重补泻、缓急补泻、迎随补泻、择向补泻。一般认为，作用时间较长的轻刺激手法可以兴奋脏器生理功能，具有"补法"的作用，而作用时间较短的重刺激手法能抑制脏器生理功能，具有"泻法"的作用。三字经流派小儿推拿以线状穴位为主，向心推为补，离心推为泻（唯有天河水穴例外），而点状穴位左右旋转次数相同，避免了临床左右补泻问题的争议。

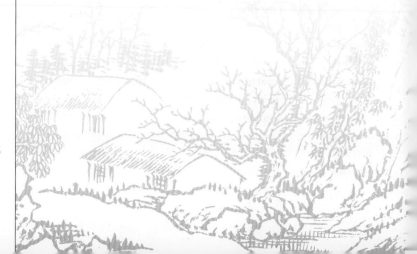

direction) along spleen-meridian point is nourishing manipulation, and pushing down (centrifugal direction) along stomach-meridian point is clearing manipulation. Pushing up (centripetal direction) *Sanguan* point has the function of ascending *yang* and nourishing *qi*, and pushing down (centrifugal direction) six-*fu* point has the function of clearing heat and expelling evil.

1.3   Reinforcing deficiency and reducing excess

Massage can be applied to reinforce deficiency and reduce excess. For deficiency syndrome, the nourishing point can be selected to enhance the function of *zang-fu organs*, increase their excitability. It is called tonifying manipulation. For example, for diarrhea due to spleen deficiency, tonifying manipulation on the spleen-meridian point strongly can restore the function of lucidity-ascending and transportation and transformation of the spleen and stomach. For excess syndrome, the point with the effect of eliminating evil can be selected to inhibit the function of *zang-fu organs*, reduce their excitability. It is called reducing manipulation. For example, for diarrhea due to damp-heat, clearing manipulation on the large-intestine-meridian point strongly can eliminate damp-heat and restore the normal bowel movement.

The reinforcing and reducing manipulation can be categorized as light-heavy reinforcing and reducing manipulation, slow-quick reinforcing and reducing manipulation, and directional reinforcing and reducing manipulation according to the strength, time, frequency and direction of the manipulation. It is generally considered that the manipulation with a longer duration and light stimulation can excite the physiological function of the organ and has the effect of reinforcing manipulation while one with a shorter duration and heavy stimulation can inhibit the physiological function of the organ and has the effect of reducing manipulation. The points of three-character-scripture school pediatric massage are mainly linear points. Centrifugal pushing manipulation on the linear points except heaven-river-water point has the function of clearing while centripetal pushing manipulation is nourishing. For dotty points, however, the duration of rotation manipulation to the left is equal to the one to the right. The dispute regarding the left-right reinforcing and reducing manipulation is avoided clinically.

4. 推拿温清有别

推拿可以温散寒邪，又可以清热散邪。推拿调节寒热，一是通过不同的穴位来体现，二是手法上温清有别。穴位可分为暖穴，即具有推动人体产热的功能，扶正气的穴位，如外劳宫穴可以温阳散寒，升阳举陷，治疗一切虚寒证；一窝风穴可以发散风寒，宣通表里，可以治疗伤风感冒、腹痛等；凉穴，即具有加强人体的散热功能的穴位，如推六腑穴可以清实火，退高热，对于便秘、痢疾均可以应用；天河水穴可以清热解表、泻心火。

二、小儿的生理、病理、病因特点

小儿从出生到成年，处于不断生长发育的过程中，无论在生理、病理等方面都有其自身的特点和规律，年龄越小越显著。归纳起来，其生理特点主要表现为脏腑娇嫩，形气未充；生机蓬勃，发育迅速。病理特点主要表现为发病容易，传变迅速；脏气清灵，易趋康复。正确认识和掌握小儿生理病理特点，对了解小儿生长发育、预防保健和疾病发生、发展及诊治均有极其重要的指导意义。

1. 生理特点

脏腑娇嫩，形气未充　脏腑即五脏六腑。娇，指娇气，不耐寒暑；嫩，指嫩弱。形，指形体结构，即四肢百骸、筋肉骨骼、精血津液等；气，指生理功能活动，如肺气、脾气、肾气等。充，即充实。脏腑娇嫩，形气未充，即小儿时期机体各系统和器官的形态发育及生理功能都处在不成熟和不完善的阶段。

1.4 The difference between warm-manipulation and cold-manipulation in massage

Massage has the functions of either warming and dissipating cold or clearing and dispersing heat. It adjusts cold and heat conditions by selecting different points and manipulations. Some points pertain to warm points which can promote the heat-producing function of the human body and reinforce healthy *qi*. For example, dorsal-*laogong* point has the functions of warming *yang* to dissipate cold, and elevating *yang* to raise the drooping and is used to treat deficiency syndrome. *Yiwofeng* point has the function of dispersing wind and cold, and relieving exterior and interior syndromes and is used to treat cold and abdominal pain. Cold points, however, can increase the function of heat-dispersing. For example, pushing six-*fu* point can be applied to the treatment of both constipation and dysentery by its function of clearing excessive fire and relieving high heat. Heaven-river-water point has the effect of clearing away heat and releasing exterior, and purging heart fire.

2 Physiological, Pathological and Etiological Characteristics of Children

Children are growing and developing constantly from birth to adulthood and they have their own characteristics and regular pattern in the physiological and pathological aspects. The younger, the more significant. In a word, their physiological characteristics mainly cover delicate organs, immature physique and *qi*, full of vigor, and rapid development. Their pathological characteristics mainly include falling ill easily, changing rapidly, and rehabilitating easily because of their keen visceral *qi*. Understanding and grasping the mentioned-above characteristics correctly has great significance for the understanding of children's growth and development, health care and disease prevention as well as the occurrence, development, diagnosis and treatment of disease.

2.1 Physiological characteristics

Delicate organs and immature physique and *qi* (*xing qi wei chong*):
Zang-fu means five *zang*-organs and six *fu*-organs. Delicate means tender, weak, and cold and heat intolerance. *Xing* implies physique and structure, namely

　　小儿的生理特点，历代医家有较多的论述。清代吴鞠通经过长期临床观察，认为小儿时期的机体柔嫩、气血未充、脾胃薄弱、肾气未充、腠理疏松、神气怯弱、筋骨未坚等特点是"稚阴稚阳"的表现。现代中医儿科界认为："稚阴稚阳"既是小儿的生理特点，也是小儿病理基础，由于"稚阳"的存在，某些脏腑在功能上表现相对不足，如"脾常不足"，在临床上表现为易患消化不良；由于"稚阴"的存在，某些脏腑"阴"相对不足而出现"阳"的有余，如"肝常有余"，在临床上容易出现高热惊厥；而生理特点是前提，没有"稚阴稚阳"的生理特点，就不会伴有"肝常有余，脾常不足"的病理特点。

　　生机蓬勃，发育迅速　生机，指生命力、活力；生机蓬勃，发育迅速，是指小儿在生长发育过程中，无论在机体的形态结构方面，还是各种生理功能活动方面，都是在迅速地、不断地向着成熟完善方面发展。年龄越小，这种发育的速度愈快，古代医家把小儿生机蓬勃、发育迅速的特点概括为"纯阳之体"。"纯阳"并非有阳无阴，而是指小儿生机旺盛以及对水谷精气、营养物质的需求，相对而言更加迫切，"纯阳"之"阳"代表生机。

　　现代中医儿科界认为，"纯阳"揭示了小儿时期生机蓬勃、发育迅速的生理特点，从整体上说明了小儿机体不断完善的过程。从"纯阳"分析小儿病理特点：① 内伤疾病少：小儿乃纯阳之体，其元气元精虽不盛，但无衰败之机，且纯阳用事，少有七情六欲、劳倦过度等病因，故内伤疾病少。② 发热性疾病多：小儿肌肤薄，藩篱疏，易感外邪，外邪入侵，阳气首先表现出抗邪能力，阳气抗邪的特点是温热、向上的，故最易出现发热，甚至高热、惊厥。③ 阳、热、实证多见：小儿为纯阳之体，以阳为用，阳盛则易化热。当外邪侵袭或内郁时，邪正相争，易患热性病证，且患病之气又易从热化，在疾病的早期出现阳、热、实证的症状。④ 疾病后期多气阴两亏：小儿乃纯阳之体，感邪后化热化火迅速，火热之邪燔灼津液，致阴液匮乏。

limbs, joints, muscles and skeletons, essence, blood, body fluid and so on. *Qi* means physical activities, such as *qi* of the lung, spleen, kidney and so on. *Wei chong* means immature. What "delicate organs and immature physique and *qi*" means is that the morphological development and physiological functions of body systems and organs in childhood are in an immature and imperfect stage.

Physiological characteristics of children have been discussed by doctors in ancient times. After long-term clinical observation, *Wu Jutong*, a noted doctor living in *Qing* Dynasty, thought that the characteristics such as delicate organism, immature *qi* and blood, weak spleen and stomach, immature kidney *qi*, loose striae and interstice, weak spirit, unsubstantial tendon and bones and so on in childhood pertained to the manifestations of "immature *yin* and *yang*" (*zhi yin zhi yang*). Modern TCM pediatrics holds that "immature *yin* and *yang*" (*zhi yin zhi yang*) is either the physiological characteristics or the pathological basis in children. The function of some *zang-fu* organs is insufficient relatively because of the existence of "immature *yang*" (*zhi yang*), for instance, the function of the spleen is insufficient, so children are clinically susceptible to indigestion. *Yang* is excessive while *yin* is insufficient relatively caused by the existence of "immature *yin*" (*zhi yin*), for instance, the liver is often in excessive condition, so children are clinically liable to high fever and convulsion. Physiological characteristics are premise. If there were no physiological characteristics of "immature *yin* and *yang*" (*zhi yin zhi yang*), there would be no pathological characteristics of "the liver is often in excessive condition and the function of the spleen is insufficient".

Full of vigor and rapid development: What "full of vigor and rapid development" means is that either the physique and structure or a variety of physiological activities in children develop rapidly and constantly toward mature and perfect condition. The younger, the more rapidly. This characteristic was generalized as "pure-*yang* constitution". "Pure-*yang*" is not *yang* without *yin*. *Yang* represents vitality, and "pure-*yang*" means exuberant vitality and relatively urgent needs to essence of water and grain and nutrients.

Modern TCM pediatrics holds that "pure-*yang*" reveals the children's physiology marked by full of vigor and rapid development and reflects the continuous improvement process of the children's body as a whole. The pediatric pathological characteristics are analyzed from the viewpoint of

31

2．病理特点

发病容易，传变迅速　小儿脏腑娇嫩，形气未充，稚阴稚阳，机体和功能均较脆弱，对疾病的抵抗力较差，加之小儿寒暖不能自调，乳食不知自节，一旦调护失宜，外则易为六淫所侵，内则易为饮食所伤，而得病之后，外邪容易深入，伤害脏腑，传变迅速。

《小儿药证直诀·原序》指出："脏腑柔弱，易虚易实，易寒易热。"这充分说明了小儿脏腑柔弱的生理特点，即决定了"易虚易实""易寒易热"的病理变化。"易虚易实"是指小儿一旦患病，邪气易实而正气易虚，实证往往可以迅速转化为虚证，或出现虚实并见、寒热错杂的证候。如小儿感冒后，可迅速发展为肺炎喘嗽，如不及时救治更容易发展为内闭外脱之危证；又如饮食不当，内伤乳食发生腹泻，不及时救治，可由实证传变为液脱阴伤，甚至亡阴亡阳之候。总之，小儿寒热虚实的变化，比成人更为迅速而错综复杂。

"pure-*yang*" as follows: ① Fewer endogenous diseases: Children have "pure-*yang* constitution". Although their original *qi* and essence is immature, there is no decline. Additionally, children are seldom attacked by such causes of diseases as seven emotions and six sensory pleasures and excessive overstrain, and therefore suffer seldom from endogenous diseases. ② More febrile diseases: Children's skin is thin and easy to be attacked by exogenous pathogenic evils. When those evils invade body, *yang qi* fights them at first. Because the characteristics of *yang qi* in fighting evils are warm and upward, fever and high fever and convulsion develop most easily. ③ *Yang*, heat, and excess syndromes are commonly seen: The body of children belongs to "pure-*yang*" constitution and its *yang* is reflected in function, *yang* exuberance is easy to cause heat. When exogenous pathogenic evils invade or stagnate interiorly, pathogenic evils and healthy *qi* fight each other, and people are liable to febrile diseases and the evils are easily transformed into heat resulting in *yang*, heat, and excess syndromes at the early stage of diseases. ④ Both *qi* and *yin* deficiency at the late stage of diseases: Because children have "pure-*yang*" constitution, the evils after invading body are rapidly transformed into heat and fire which consume the body fluid leading to deficiency of *yin*-fluid.

2.2 Pathological characteristics

Being liable to diseases, and diseases change quickly: Children have delicate organs, immature physique and *qi*, immature *yin* and *yang*, their organisms and functions are both relatively fragile and have poor resistance to diseases. In addition, children cannot adjust properly their clothes-wearing, and food-intaking by themselves. Once adjusting and nursing are given improperly, they are exteriorly prone to six exogenous evils and interiorly injured by milk and food. Once children have got an illness, exogenous evils go deep into the body easily, and hurt *zang-fu* organs, pathogenesis transmission is rapid.

In the preface of *Key to Medicines and Patterns of Children's Diseases (Xiao Er Yao Zheng Zhi Jue)*, it stated that children's *zang-fu* organs are delicate, prone to excess syndrome and deficiency syndrome, cold syndrome and heat syndrome. This fully shows that the physiological characteristics of children determine the pathological characteristics of "Being prone to deficiency syndrome and excess syndrome". The phrase

脏气清灵，易趋康复 小儿疾病在病情发展转归过程中，由于生理上生机旺盛，发育迅速，活力充沛，患病以后容易恢复，这是有利条件；小儿的病理有寒热虚实易变，病情易恶化的一方面；但其生机蓬勃，组织再生和修补的过程较快，且病因比较单纯，在疾病过程中又少七情影响，所以轻病容易治愈，重病若治疗及时，护理得宜，病情比成人好转得快，容易恢复健康。

3. 病因特点

小儿疾病发生的原因基本上与成人相同，但小儿具有脏腑娇嫩，形气未充，卫外功能未固，正气不足的体质特点，因此在发病上对许多时行疾病如风疹、幼儿急疹、流行性腮腺炎、百日咳、水痘等有特殊的易感性，且为小儿时期多见或特有。

小儿病因较成人单纯，外多感于六淫，内多伤于乳食，故肺系和脾胃病证多见。还有一些小儿因先天不足，后天失养而患有五迟、五软、解颅等特有病证。此外，智识未开，缺乏生活知识，每因看护不周，易发生跌仆损伤、烫伤、刀伤、溺水、触电、中毒等意外事故。综上所述，小儿在病因方面有先天因素、外感因素、内伤因素及意外因素等较为多见的特点。

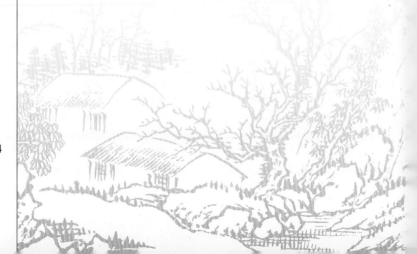

means that the evils easily cause excess syndrome, the healthy *qi* easily becomes deficient, and the excess syndrome may often transformed into deficiency syndrome or deficiency-excess in complexity syndrome and cold-heat in complexity syndrome once children get illness. If a child catches a cold, for instance, he is rapidly prone to develop dyspnea and cough due to pneumonia, and the latter will more easily become critical syndrome of internal block and external collapse once emergency measures are not taken in time. If a baby with diarrhea caused by improper diet doesn't get a timely treatment, the syndrome will change from excess syndrome to fluid-collapse and *yin*-injury, and *yin* exhaustion and *yang* exhaustion syndrome. In a word, the change of children in cold-heat-deficiency-excess syndrome is quicker and more complicated than adults'.

Clear, keen visceral *qi* and recovering easily: When children are ill, they recover easily because of their exuberance, rapid development, and full of vigor in physiology. This is advantage. Children's disease change quickly in cold-heat-deficiency-excess aspect and their conditions become worse easily but they have exuberance, quicker tissue regeneration and repair process, simple etiology, and less emotional impact and therefore children with light disease heal easily and children with heavy disease recover more quickly than adults if timely treatment and proper nursing are given.

2.3 Etiological characteristics

The children's etiology is basically the same as the adults'. Having their special physical characteristics, however, children are especially prone to many epidemic diseases such as rubella, infantile acute rash, mumps, whooping cough, chicken pox and so on which are commonly-seen or unique in children.

The etiology of children is simpler than adults', and children are mostly prone to the diseases caused by six exogenous factors exteriorly and to the ones caused by milk and food. So lung related diseases, spleen and stomach diseases are common in children. Some specific diseases such as five retardation, five kinds of flaccidity in infants, and infantile ununited skull and so on occur in some children who are congenitally deficient and lack of acquired nutrients. In addition, accidents such as fall and injury, scald, cuts, drowning, electric shock, and poisoning happen easily. The reason for this is because children are lack of knowledge of life and have got loose care. In summary, the causes of diseases in children mainly cover congenital, exogenous, endogenous, and unexpected factors and so on.

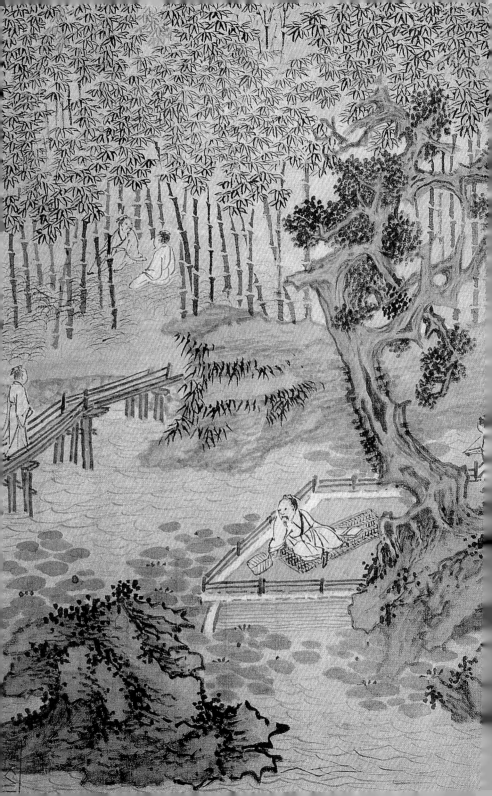

一、推拿手法

三字经流派小儿推拿手法简单易学，常用的只有6种手法。

1. 推法

该法是在穴位上用拇指桡侧面或示指、中指螺纹面做直线推动，也就是有规律地、轻重均匀地连续直线摩擦称为推法（图3-1）。一般离心的方向为清，向心的方向为补，来回往复为清补。推法用于线状的穴位。

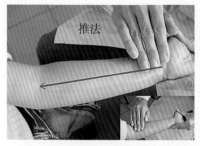

图3-1　推法
Picture 3-1　Pushing

2. 揉法

该法以医者的手指按在操作的穴位上，不离其处而旋转揉动称为揉法（图3-2）。一般是用拇指或中示两指的掌面揉之，左揉右揉同数，左揉主升，右揉主降，其作用多偏于补，也含有清补的作用。揉法用于点状的穴位。

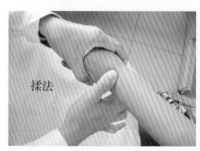

图3-2　揉法
Picture 3-2　Kneading

3. 拿法

该法以拇、示两指或并用中指，夹住穴位同时用力，一紧一松，反复增减用力称为拿法（图3-3）。本派拿法专用于列缺穴，是一种刺激强烈的手法。

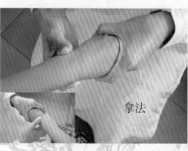

图3-3　拿法
Picture 3-3　Grasping

1 Manipulations

Simple and easy, this school of massage has only six main manipulations.

1.1 Pushing

Regularly, evenly and continuously, push the point straight by using your radial side of thumb or the joint fingerprint surfaces of index and middle fingers. (Picture 3 – 1) Usually, centrifugal pushing has the function of clearing while centripetal pushing is nourishing. In addition, to-and-fro pushing is harmonizing. This manipulation is applied to linear points.

1.2 Kneading

Press your finger (fingerprint surface of thumb or index and middle fingers) on the point; knead it without removing the finger. (Picture 3 – 2) Kneading to both sides (right and left) should be equal. Left kneading governs ascending and right, descending. In general, the nourishing function of kneading overweighs clearing function. Also, the function has some proportion of harmonizing. This manipulation is applied to dotty points.

1.3 Grasping

Grasp and release the point in turn by using your thumb and index finger or adding the middle finger. (Picture 3 – 3) Grasping in our school is specialized in *lieque* point and it is a manipulation with strong stimulation.

4．捣法

医者的中指或示指屈曲，以其屈指关节背面捣在穴位处称为捣法（图3-4）。捣法用于点状穴位。

5．分合法

用医者两大拇指的外侧同时从穴位处向两旁分推为分法，同时从穴位两边向穴位处合推为合法（图3-5）。分合法用于线状穴位。

6．运法

用医者拇指侧面或示指、中指、无名指并拢的螺纹面，循穴位向一定方向转整圈回环摩动，或做弧形推动称为运法（图3-6）。

二、推拿的润滑剂

推拿时连续摩擦，因皮肤出汗，必然滞涩而不流畅，既不便于推运，且容易发炎，必须用润滑剂助之。旧法葱水、姜水、香油、冬青油等，具有帮助通透的作用。推拿是否有效还是在于摩擦，旧法所用之物爽滑力不大，反而湿腻不快，而滑石细粉，干爽滑利，久推无碍，比旧法便利许多，特别是采用"独穴"多推，更为适用。因此，三字经流派小儿推拿介质只用滑石粉。

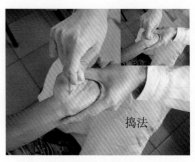

图3-4　捣法
Picture 3-4　Pounding

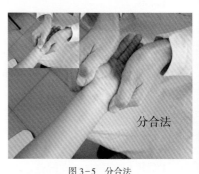

图3-5　分合法
Picture 3-5　Parting-pushing and Meeting-pushing

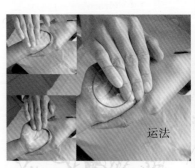

图3-6　运法
Picture 3-6　Arc-pushing

1.4 Pounding

Flex your middle or index finger and use the knuckle to pound the point. (Picture 3 – 4) This manipulation is used for dotty points.

1.5 Parting-pushing and meeting-pushing

Parting-pushing: put your thumbs on the point and part them by pushing to each own side at an appropriate distance.

Meeting-pushing: put your thumbs a certain distance away from the point at each side, and meet them by pushing towards the point. (Picture 3 – 5) This manipulation is used for linear points.

1.6 Arc-pushing

Repeatedly and in one direction, push the point around or in an arch by using your lateral side of thumb or the palmar surfaces of index, middle and third fingers. (Picture 3 – 6)

2　Lubricant Used in Massage

In the course of massage, continuous manipulation induces sweating. Inevitably, sweat sticks to the skin, which is not only bad for smooth manipulation, but also easy to get inflamed. So, a lubricant is required. In old times, lubricants such as green Chinese onion juice solution, ginger juice solution, sesame oil and Chinese holly oil were used. They are effective at penetrating but too greasy for manipulating. In fact, effectiveness of massage lies in the friction. For this, doctor *Li Dexiu*, selected talcum fine powder as the lubricant. The talcum fine powder is dry and smooth, which is good for manipulation for a long time and much more convenient than the ancient lubricants. It is especially suitable to be adopted in a single point for manipulation for a long time.

三、常用穴位

推拿得效，手法的正确和穴位的准确都是首要的。徐氏的原著并无刊行本，经多人传抄摹写，穴位图多已失真，说明也欠明了。下文以王蕴华整理的《李德修小儿推拿技法》（1981年青岛市中医院印）为依据，因头面穴位很少用之，在此不做介绍，也不征引其他推拿流派的资料。

1. 心经穴

部位　中指掌面，由指尖到指根，属线状穴位。（图3-7）

手法　一般用清补法。本穴在临床上极少用，如有心火，也不得用清法，而以推天河水代之。

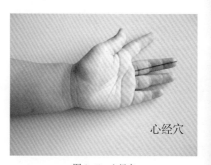

图3-7　心经穴
Picture 3-7　Heart-meridian point

2. 肝经穴

部位　示指掌面，由指尖到指根，属线状穴位。（图3-8）

手法　一般用清法，习惯上称为平肝。其清法则是从示指根部之横纹起一直推到指尖，此穴非肝极虚不能妄用补法。

主治　发热、感冒、烦躁不安、头晕头痛。此外，肝气郁结、神志抑郁，也可以专用平肝法，功效同于方剂的"逍遥散"。

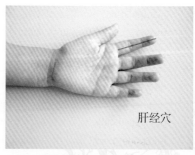

图3-8　肝经穴
Picture 3-8　Liver-meridian point

3 Main Points

An effective massage should give priority to correct manipulations and accurate points. *Xu*'s original paper was not published but available for reference purposes. Moreover, the pictures of the points were anamorphic and comments were unclear. Points in this article are solely based on *Li Dexiu* Massage Manipulation for Pediatrics, a book compiled by *Wang Yunhua* and printed by *Qingdao* TCM Hospital in 1981. Points in head are seldom to be selected in clinic and no introduction is provided here.

3.1 Heart-meridian point
• It is a linear point along the ventral side of the middle finger, from its tip to root. (Picture 3 – 7)
• In manipulation, push this point to and fro. But this point is seldom adopted in clinic because pushing heaven-river-water point is much more effective to clear heart fire.

3.2 Liver-meridian point
• It is a linear point along the ventral side of the index finger, from its tip to root. (Picture 3 – 8)
• This point is mainly used for clearing, also referred as pacifying liver. In manipulation, push the index finger straight from the transverse crease of its root to the tip for clearing. No nourishing manipulation is applied to this point except when the liver is extremely deficient.
• It is used for treating fever, common cold, fidgeting, dizziness and headache. In addition, pacifying liver has equivalent curative effect to the prescription of *Xiaoyao* Powder for treating stagnation of liver *qi* and depression.

43

3. 脾经穴

部位 拇指外侧,由指尖到指根,属线状穴位。(图3-9)

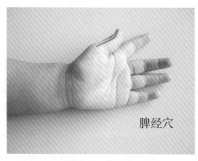

脾经穴

图3-9 脾经穴
Picture 3-9 Spleen-meridian point

手法 屈指向心推之为补(不屈亦可),屈指离心推之为清,来回推之为清补。

主治 脾虚作泻,先清补大肠以止泻。然后清补脾以加强消化健运。

大便燥结伸大指向外推之,以泻其火,再用泻大肠法,燥结可愈,后用补肾法以善其后。

心脾火盛,口舌生疮,手热身热,先推天河水,然后清补脾。

唇裂肿痛,口外生疮,上眼皮肿,皆属脾火,也有因虚寒而肿的,一律用清补脾法通治。

4. 肺经穴

部位 无名指掌面,由指尖到指根,属线状穴位。(图3-10)

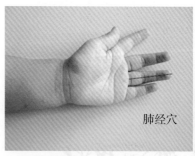

肺经穴

图3-10 肺经穴
Picture 3-10 Lung-meridian point

手法 清法则从无名指根部之横纹起一直推到指尖,补法从无名指端推到指根,但补法少用。

主治 清肺法常与平肝、推天河水配合应用,以退热。肺非极虚不宜妄补,若欲补肺,可用补脾法以代之。

3.3 Spleen-meridian point

• It is a linear point along the lateral side of the thumb, from its tip to root. (Picture 3 – 9)

• In manipulation, let the patient flex (or not) the thumb. Centrifugal pushing has the function of clearing while centripetal pushing is nourishing, and to-and-fro is harmonizing.

• For diarrhea due to spleen deficiency, push large-intestine-meridian point to and fro to relieve diarrhea first. Then push spleen-meridian point to and fro to promote the function of transportation and transformation.

For dry and hard stool, push centrifugally on spleen-meridian point to clear heat first, then push large-intestine-meridian point for purging. After recovery, nourish the kidney-meridian point to rehabilitate.

For intense heat in the heart and spleen with symptoms as aphtha, tongue sores, feverish sensation in the body and hands, push heaven-river-water point first, and then push spleen-meridian point to and fro.

For sore, swelled and chapped lips, aphtha and swollen upper eyelids induced by spleen fire or deficiency-cold, push spleen-meridian point to and fro overall.

3.4 Lung-meridian point

• It is a linear point in the ventral side of the third finger, from its tip to root. (Picture 3 – 10)

• In manipulation, push the third finger straight from the transverse crease of its root to tip for clearing and in opposite direction for nourishing. This point is seldom selected for nourishing.

• For clearing heat, it is common to use both the liver-meridian point and heaven-river-water point. No nourishing manipulation is applied to this point except when the lung is extremely deficient. If nourishment is needed, substitute splenic nourishment for it.

5. 肾经穴

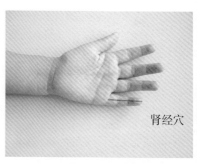

肾经穴

图 3-11　肾经穴
Picture 3-11　Kidney-meridian point

部位　小指掌面，由指尖到指根，属线状穴位。（图3-11）

手法　从小指端推到指根部为补法，不用清法。

主治　肾水不足，则虚火上炎，非一般清热法所能降，必须用补肾法以滋肾水，则虚火自退。

肝不宜补，肝虚者，用补肾法生肾水以养肝，即为补肝。

6. 小肠经穴

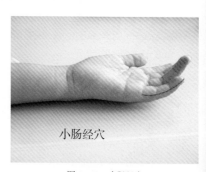

小肠经穴

图 3-12　小肠经穴
Picture 3-12　Small-intestine-meridian point

部位　小指外侧，由指尖到指根，属线状穴位。（图3-12）

手法　小指外侧从指根到指尖为清，来回推为清补，不用补法。

主治　膀胱气化不行，则小便不利，须用清法以化郁行气。

小肠能分水液别清浊，用清补法，可以利水道而通小便。

3.5　Kidney-meridian point

• It is a linear point along the ventral side of the little finger, from its tip to root. (Picture 3 – 11)

• In manipulation, push the ventral side of the little finger straight from the tip to the transverse crease of the root for nourishing. No clearing manipulation on this point.

• For kidney *yin* deficiency with deficient fire, heat-clearing treatment is of no effect and kidney nourishment must be adopted to replenish kidney *yin* and thus deficiency-fire is repelled.

• For liver deficiency, as the liver is not recommended to be nourished directly, nourish kidney to replenish kidney *yin* and by water moistening wood, liver is reinforced.

3.6　Small-intestine-meridian point

• It is a linear point along the lateral side of the little finger, from its tip to root. (Picture 3 – 12)

• In manipulation, push the lateral side of the little finger straight from the tip to the transverse crease of its root for nourishing while to-and-fro for its harmonizing. No nourishing manipulation on this point.

• For dysuria caused by the failure of *qi* transformation of bladder, the therapeutic principle is relieving stagnation and moving *qi* by clearing small intestine.

The function of small intestine is isolating the essence from the turbid, and so by pushing small intestine meridian point to and fro, it has the function of regulating water channel to induce urine.

7. 胃经穴

部位 大鱼际外缘赤白肉际处，自腕横纹到拇指根部，属线状穴位。（图3-13）

手法 自大鱼际外缘赤白肉际处，从腕横纹推至拇指根部为清法；反之则为补法。清之则气下降，补之则气上升。因胃气以息息下行为顺，一般用清法。

主治 清胃热，降胃气，一般呕吐皆可用之。胃气下降而不上逆，呕吐可愈。

8. 板门穴

部位 掌面大鱼际正中，属点状穴位。（图3-14）

手法 按住大鱼际正中，左右旋揉同数。

主治 脾胃虚实所致上吐下泻皆可揉之。

9. 大肠经穴

部位 示指外侧，由指尖到指根，属线状穴位。（图3-15）

手法 由示指外侧从指根到指尖推为清，向虎口方向推为补，来回推为清补，一般不专用补法。

主治 清则气下降，补则气上升，清补则和血顺气。泄泻痢疾，用清补法，多推此一穴可愈。

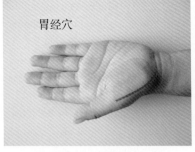

图3-13 胃经穴
Picture 3-13 Stomach-meridian point

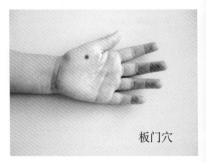

图3-14 板门穴
Picture 3-14 *Banmen* point

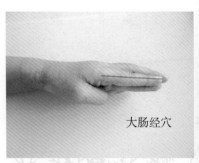

图3-15 大肠经穴
Picture 3-15 Large-intestine-meridian point

3.7   Stomach-meridian point

• It is a linear point in the dorso-ventral boundary of the lateral side of the big thenar from transverse crease of the wrist to the root of the thumb. (Picture 3 – 13)

• In manipulation, push this point from transverse crease of the wrist to the root of the thumb for clearing while in opposite direction for nourishing. By clearing, *qi* tends to descend and by nourishing, *qi* tends to ascend. Stomach *qi* is descendent in physiology, so clearing therapy is much more common to be adopted here.

• It has the function of clearing stomach heat and checking adverse rising of stomach *qi*, and thus it is used for treating common vomiting. If stomach *qi* descends and does not ascend, there will be no vomiting.

3.8   *Banmen* point

• It is a dotty point in the middle of the big thenar. (Picture 3 – 14)

• In manipulation, press this point and knead it. Kneading to both sides (right and left) should be equal.

• It is used for treating vomiting and diarrhea caused by deficiency or excess of the spleen and stomach.

3.9   Large-intestine-meridian point

• It is a linear point along the lateral side of the index finger, from its tip to root. (Picture 3 – 15)

• In manipulation, push this point straight from the finger root to the tip for clearing while in opposite direction, for nourishing, and to and fro, for harmonizing. Usually, no nourishing manipulation is solely adopted.

• *Qi* is descendant by clearing, ascendant by nourishing and regulated by harmonizing. Also, blood circulation is smoothed through harmonizing therapy. For diarrhea and dysentery, it is quite effective to push this point to and fro for a long duration.

10．四横纹穴

部位　示指、中指、无名指、小指连掌之纹，属线状穴位。（图3-16）

手法　来回推之。

主治　开脏腑寒热，治腹胀；揉之，能和气血。

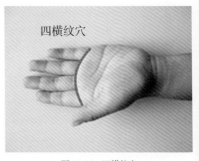

四横纹穴

图3-16　四横纹穴
Picture 3-16　Four-transverse-crease point

11．小天心穴

部位　在掌根，大小鱼际交接之中点凹陷中，属点状穴位。（图3-17）

手法　用捣法，上下左右捣或直捣，随症采用。

主治　镇静安神，主治惊风。

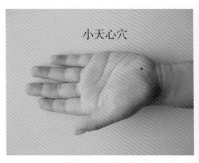

小天心穴

图3-17　小天心穴
Picture 3-17　Small-heaven-center point

12．小横纹穴

部位　小指与掌相连之纹下又一横纹，穴在尺侧掌纹头，属点状穴位。（图3-18）

手法　揉之左右同数。

主治　治咳嗽。

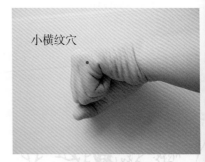

小横纹穴

图3-18　小横纹穴
Picture 3-18　Little-transverse-crease point

3.10 Four-transverse-crease point

- It is a linear point with the whole line of the transverse crease of the finger root of the index, middle, third and little fingers. (Picture 3 – 16)
- In manipulation, push it to and fro.
- It has the function of regulating visceral heat and cold, and thus it is used for treating distension in abdomen.

If kneading manipulation is applied to this point, it is capable of harmonizing *qi* and blood.

3.11 Small-heaven-center point

- It is a dotty point in the dent at the intersection of the small and big thenars. (Picture 3 – 17)
- In manipulation, pound the point. According to symptoms, there will be different pounding manipulations, such as slant pounding and vertical pounding.
- It has the function of inducing sedation and tranquilization, and thus it is used for treating infantile convulsions.

3.12 Little-transverse-crease point

- It is a dotty point in the ulnar side of the first transverse crease of the palm below the little finger. (Picture 3 – 18)
- In manipulation, knead it. Kneading amounts of both sides (right and left) should be equal.
- It is used for treating cough.

13. 八卦穴

部位 在手掌面，以掌心为圆心，从圆心至中指根横纹约 2/3 处为半径，画一圆圈，此圆即为八卦穴。（图 3-19）

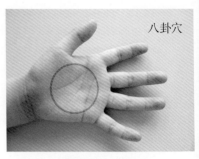

图 3-19 八卦穴
Picture 3-19 *Bagua* point

手法 用运法，顺时针方向为顺运八卦；反之为逆运八卦。

主治 五脏之气不调而胸膈作闷、痰火郁结、喘嗽交作、小儿百日咳等，均可用运八卦法，以宽胸利膈，且能加强中气的运化力量，以消痞化积。咳嗽气逆者逆运八卦，以降肺气。

14. 分阴阳穴

部位 掌根部，小天心穴两侧，属线状穴位。（图 3-20）

手法 从小天心穴向两侧分推。

主治 分寒热，平气血，寒热错综，气血不和，病变复杂，用此法以解寒热，使气血舒和。

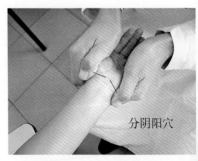

图 3-20 分阴阳穴
Picture 3-20 Parting-*yin-yang* point

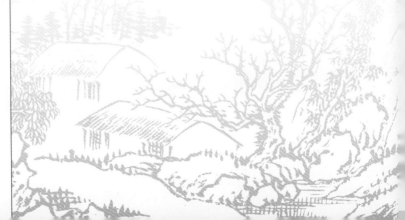

3.13 *Bagua* point

• It is a circle point with the center of palm as its center and 2/3 of the center to the transverse crease of the middle finger root as the radius. (Picture 3 – 19)

• In manipulation, arc-push this point clockwise or counter-clockwise.

• It has the function of soothing chest and benefiting diaphragm, and thus it is used for treating oppression in chest, phlegm-fire accumulation, repeated cough, infantile whooping cough, which are caused by disharmony *qi* of five *zang*-organs. Also, it is able to strengthen transportation force of *qi* in the middle-*jiao* to resolve stuffiness and food stagnation. For cough due to reversed flow of *qi*, arc-push this point counter-clockwise to direct lung *qi* downward.

3.14 Parting-*yin-yang* point

• It is a linear point at the root of palm and by the two sides of the small-heaven-center point. (Picture 3 – 20)

• In manipulation, parting-push from small-heaven-center point to opposite side.

• It has the function of distinguishing heat and cold, harmonizing *qi* and blood, and thus it is used for treating intricate diseases caused by interweaved cold-heat, as well as *qi* and blood in disharmony.

15．合阴阳穴

部位 掌根部，小天心穴两侧，属线状穴位。（图3-21）

手法 与分阴阳方向相反，从两侧向中心推之。

主治 徐氏用本法与他穴配合治痰涎壅盛，其法先推肾经穴，次用合阴阳经，最后推天河水，其痰即散。

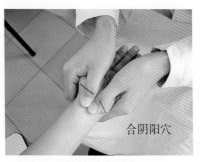

图3-21 合阴阳穴
Picture 3-21 Meeting-*yin-yang* point

16．运水入土穴

部位 自小指尖沿掌边推向拇指根，属弧形穴位。（图3-22）

手法 做弧形推动。

主治 便秘，亦可治遗尿。

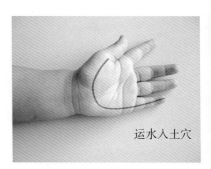

图3-22 运水入土穴
Picture 3-22 Water-to-earth point

17．运土入水穴

部位 自拇指尖沿掌边推向小指根，属弧形穴位。（图3-23）

手法 做弧形推动。

主治 腹泻。

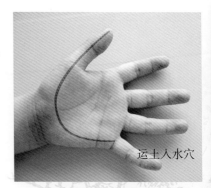

图3-23 运土入水穴
Picture 3-23 Earth-to-water point

3.15 Meeting-*yin-yang* point

- It is a linear point at the root of palm and by the two sides of the small-heaven-center point. (Picture 3 – 21)
- In manipulation, meeting-push from opposite sides to small-heaven-center point, just opposite to the direction of manipulation on parting-*yin-yang* point.
- This point is often combined with other points to treat phlegm-fluid retention. The method is as follows: push kidney-meridian point first, then meeting-push meeting-*yin-yang* point, and push heaven-river-water point at last.

3.16 Water-to-earth point

- It is an arc-point from the tip of little finger to the root of thumb. (Picture 3 – 22)
- In manipulation, arc-push this point from the tip of little finger to the root of thumb.
- It is used for treating constipation, and also enuresis.

3.17 Earth-to-water point

- It is an arc-point from the tip of thumb to the root of the little finger. (Picture 3 – 23)
- In manipulation, arc-push this point from the tip of thumb to the root of the little finger.
- It is used for treating diarrhea.

18．天河水穴

部位　自腕横纹中央到肘横纹，属线状穴位。（图 3-24）

手法　自腕横纹中央推向肘横纹中央止。

主治　心经有热不能直接清泄，用此穴清心火，退热解表，常与平肝清肺配合。

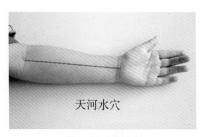

图 3-24　天河水穴
Picture 3-24　Heaven-river-water point

19．三关穴

部位　前臂桡侧面，自腕横纹到肘横纹，属线状穴位。（图 3-25）

手法　将患者左臂顺正，使拇指在上，推的部位保持在臂的上侧，自腕横纹到肘横纹，属线状穴位。

主治　此为温穴，大补肾中元气，回阳生热，主治一切虚寒证。

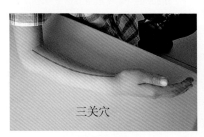

图 3-25　三关穴
Picture 3-25　*Sanguan* point

20．六腑穴

部位　前臂尺侧面，自肘横纹到腕横纹，属线状穴位。（图 3-26）

手法　将患者左臂顺正，使小指在下，推的部位保持在臂的下侧，自肘横纹到腕横纹，属线状穴位。

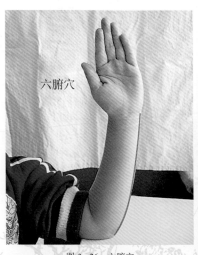

图 3-26　六腑穴
Picture 3-26　Six-*fu* point

主治　此为凉穴，亦具有壮水制火、滋阴潜阳之功，主治头目牙耳实火之证及虚火上炎之证。

3.18 Heaven-river-water point

• It is a linear point between centers of transverse crease of the wrist and the transverse crease of elbow. (Picture 3–24)

• In manipulation, push this point from the center of transverse crease of the wrist to the center of transverse crease of elbow.

• It is used for clearing heart-fire, which is improper to be cleared in heart meridian directly. For releasing exterior and discharging fire, this point is commonly combined with other points, namely pacifying liver and clearing lung-meridian point.

3.19 *Sanguan* point

• It is a linear point in the radial side of forearm from transverse crease of the wrist to the transverse crease of elbow. (Picture 3–25)

• In manipulation, keep the radial side of patient's left forearm upward and push this point from transverse crease of the wrist to that of elbow.

• It is a point for warming, which nourishes original *qi* in kidney, restores *yang* and generates heat. Thus, it is used for treating all kinds of cold-deficiency syndromes.

3.20 Six-*fu* point

• It is a linear point in the ulnar side of forearm from transverse crease of the elbow to the transverse crease of wrist. (Picture 3–26)

• In manipulation, keep the ulnar side of patient's left forearm downward and push this point from transverse crease of the elbow to the transverse crease of wrist.

• It is a point for cooling, and also for engendering water to control fire, nourishing *yin* and subduing *yang*. Thus, it is used for treating both excess and deficient fire in head, eye, tooth and ear.

21. 外劳宫穴

部位 在掌背中指、无名指两骨中间凹处，属点状穴位。（图3－27）

手法 左右揉同数，揉时应屈患者手指。

主治 此为暖穴，善治下焦寒。凡脏腑风寒冷痛，属寒久不愈，揉不计数，以愈为度。

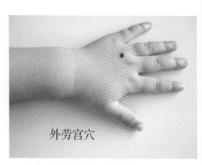

外劳宫穴

图3－27 外劳宫穴
Picture 3－27 Dorsal-*laogong* point

22. 一窝风穴

部位 在手背腕横纹正中凹陷中。（图3－28）

手法 左右揉同数。

主治 下寒腹痛，风寒鼻流清涕。

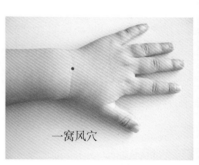

一窝风穴

图3－28 一窝风穴
Picture 3－28 *Yiwofeng* point

23. 二人上马穴

部位 本穴简称二马，在掌背小指及无名指掌指关节后凹陷处。（图3－29）

手法 左右揉同数。

主治 大补肾中水火，左揉气降右揉气升。治虚火牙痛，眼赤而不痛。一切属肾虚的症候，都可以用此穴补肾为治，也可用此穴以退虚热。

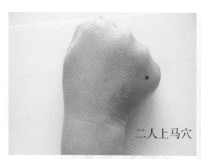

二人上马穴

图3－29 二人上马穴
Picture 3－29 *Errenshangma* point

3.21　Dorsal-*laogong* point

- It is a dotty point in the dent of dorsal side of palm between the metacarpus of the middle and third fingers. (Picture 3 – 27)
- In manipulation, keep the patient's fingers flexed and knead the point. Kneading to both sides (right and left) should be equal.
- It is a point for warming, which is good for treating cold in the lower *jiao*. Amount of kneading to this point is not specified for any wind-cold and cold pain of viscera with a long duration, the more, the better, until the recovery.

3.22　*Yiwofeng* point

- It is a dotty point of the dorsal side dent in the middle of the transverse crease of the wrist. (Picture 3 – 28)
- In manipulation, knead the point. Kneading to both sides (right and left) should be equal.
- It is used for treating cold pain in abdomen and watery nasal discharge caused by wind-cold.

3.23　*Errenshangma* point

- Abbreviated *erma*, it is a dotty point in the upper dent of the dorsal side between the third and little fingers' metacarpophalangeal joints. (Picture 3 – 29)
- In manipulation, knead the point. Kneading to both sides (right and left) should be equal.
- *Qi* tends to descend by kneading left and ascend by kneading right. This point has the function of replenishing kidney *yin* and *yang*, thus it is used for treating syndromes of kidney deficiency. Moreover, this point is used for repelling deficiency-heat, such as deficiency-fire toothache and hyperemia of eye with no pain.

24．阳池穴

部位　在手背一窝风穴上3寸，尺骨、桡骨之间即为本穴。不是针灸的阳池穴。（图3-30）

手法　左右揉同数。

主治　头部一切疾患，头痛不论寒热虚实皆效。揉不计数，以愈为度。

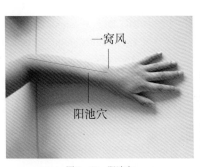

图3-30　阳池穴
Picture 3-30　*Yangchi* point

25．列缺穴

部位　在掌根连腕处两侧凹陷内，非针灸之列缺穴。（图3-31）

手法　用拇指及中指将腕窝两侧凹陷处用力卡拿，这就是推拿的"拿"法。

主治　此为出汗、解表、通窍之穴。拿之汗出为止。治伤风感冒，风寒头痛，久拿可以得汗，又可助疹痘发表，得汗后则须避风。

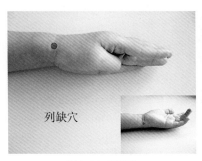

图3-31　列缺穴
Picture 3-31　*Lieque* point

26．五指节穴

部位　五指各关节。（图3-32）

手法　用指端指甲里外揉、捻、掐之。

主治　祛风、镇惊、和血、顺气，并消痞积。多用得效。诸穴推毕，都可用此法以和气血。

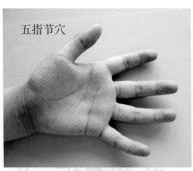

图3-32　五指节穴
Picture 3-32　Finger-knuckle point

3.24 *Yangchi* point

- This point locates 3 *cun* above *yiwofeng*, between radius and ulna. It is different from the point of *Yangchi* (TE 4/SJ 4) in acupuncture. (Picture 3-30)

- In manipulation, knead the point. Kneading to both sides (right and left) should be equal.

- It is used for treating diseases in the head. It is especially effective to headache, regardless of cold, heat, deficient and excess syndromes. Amount of kneading to this point is not specified, the more, the better, until the recovery.

2.25 *Lieque* point

- It is the two dents in the transverse crease of wrist, one on ulnar side, and another on radial side. It is not the point of *Lieque* (LU 7) in acupuncture. (Picture 3-31)

- In manipulation, grasp and release both dents of this point in turn by using your thumb and index finger.

- It has the function of inducing sweating, releasing exterior and opening orifice. Grasp the point until sweating. It is used for treating common cold and wind-cold headache. Long time of grasping manipulation is adopted to induce sweating and release exterior to promote eruption. After sweating, avoid catching wind-cold!

3.26 Finger-knuckle point

- It refers to the knuckles of the five fingers. (Picture 3-32)

- In manipulation, knead, holding-twist and pinch the knuckles by using your fingers nails

- It is effective of dispelling wind, inducing sedation, harmonizing blood, regulating *qi* movement, relieving stuffiness and removing food stagnation. In addition, it is used as the ending step of massage to harmonize *qi* and blood.

27．威灵穴

部位　手背第2～3掌骨中央之间的凹陷中。（图3-33）

手法　用指端指甲揉、掐之。

主治　与捣小天心、掐五指节、掐揉精宁穴同用，诸穴推毕，都可用此法以和气血。

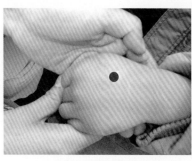

图3-33　威灵穴
Picture 3-33　*Weiling* point

28．精宁穴

部位　手背第4～5掌骨中央之间的凹陷中。（图3-34）

手法　用指端指甲揉、掐之。

主治　与捣小天心、掐五指节、掐揉威灵穴同用，诸穴推毕，都可用此法以和气血。

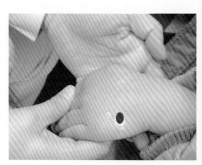

图3-34　精宁穴
Picture 3-34　*Jingning* point

以上共28个穴位，其中有的未经使用过，凡用过得效的都作了说明。三字经流派小儿推拿，概用左手，不照男左女右的旧法，其中穴位手法与其他流派资料的异同，在此不加考订。

3.27   *Weiling* point

- It is a dotty point in the dent of dorsal side of palm between the metacarpus of the second and middle fingers. (Picture 3 – 33)
- In manipulation, knead, holding-twist and pinch the knuckles by using your fingers nails.
- It is used with pounding little-transverse-crease point, kneading finger-knuckle point and *Jingning* together as the ending step of massage to harmonize *qi* and blood.

3.28   *Jingning* point

- It is a dotty point in the dent of dorsal side of palm between the metacarpus of the ring and little fingers. (Picture 3 – 34)
- In manipulation, knead, holding-twist and pinch the knuckles by using your fingers nails.
- It is used with pounding little-transverse-crease point, kneading finger-knuckle point and *Weining* together as the ending step of massage to harmonize *qi* and blood.

There are altogether 28 points here. Most of them are quite effective and are all illustrated above. In old times, manipulation is on the right hand of boy and left hand of girl. However, the manipulation of Three-character-scripture School Massage is solely on the left hand. No material is presented here to compare the difference of points and manipulations with other schools massage.

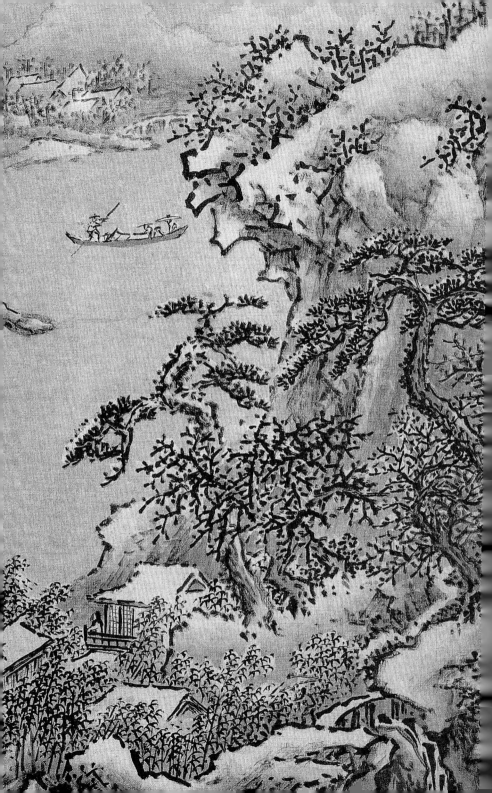

Chapter 4
Clinical Application of
Three-Character-Scripture School Massage

第四章
三字经流派小儿推拿的临床应用

本章仅介绍当前儿科推拿治疗的主要病症。三字经流派小儿推拿的特点是取穴少，每穴操作时间长，一般情况下每穴 15 分钟左右，个别病重的可到 20～30 分钟，而目前每一人次推拿总时间为 20～30 分钟，因此，小儿肺炎、痢疾等疾病已不作为推拿治疗的主要病症。

第一节　发热

发热即体温异常升高，是儿科疾病中的常见症状，正常小儿腋下体温为 36℃～37℃（口表、肛表依次高 0.3℃～0.5℃），午后体温较清晨为高，可受环境温度、进食或饥饿、活动多少、衣着厚薄、哭闹等影响而在一定范围内波动，当体温升高超过正常基础体温 1℃以上时，可诊断为发热。发热可分为低热（37.5℃～38℃）、中度发热（38.1℃～39℃）、高热（39.1℃～41℃）、过高热（＞41℃）。

病因病机
中医根据感邪性质不同将发热分为外感和内伤两大类。外感发热多因感受风寒、风热、暑热等六淫之邪，具有起病急、传变快的特点，属实证；内伤发热多有内伤病因存在，如因乳食所伤、惊恐、阴阳失调而致；病程长，热势多样，属虚证，且外感与内伤诸因素互相影响。

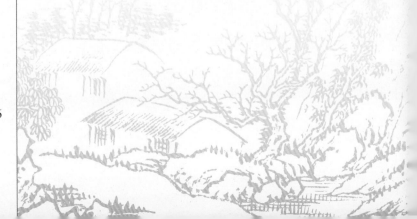

In this chapter, we will introduce some common diseases of pediatrics treated with massage. The characteristics of Three-character-scripture School Massage are fewer points for treatment and longer duration of manipulation. Usually, the duration of manipulation on each point is about 15min and 20 − 30min in severe cases. The total duration of manipulation of one patient is about 20-30min now, so some diseases such as pneumonia and dysentery have been excluded because of too long time to manipulate in clinic. We generally treat them with other methods.

Section 1　Fever

Fever is abnormal high body temperature. It is a common symptom in pediatrics. The temperature of a normal infant is 36 ℃ − 37 ℃ in armpit and 0.3 ℃ − 0.5 ℃ higher in mouth and anus. Body temperature fluctuates in a range. For example, it is higher in the afternoon than in the morning and is influenced by the environmental temperature, eating or starving, physical activities, coating, mood and so on. When the temperature excels the basic temperature to more than 1 ℃ , it is considered as fever. There are low fever (37.5 ℃ − 38 ℃), medial fever (38.1 ℃ − 39 ℃), high fever (39.1 ℃ − 41 ℃) and very high fever (>41 ℃).

Cause and mechanism of disease

According to the nature of pathogen, there are fever of external contraction and fever of internal injury in TCM. Fever of external contraction is triggered by six excesses, such as wind-cold pathogen, wind-heat pathogen and summer-heat pathogen. It is characterized as abrupt onset, fast transmission and development and belongs to excess syndrome. Fever of internal injury is caused by internal pathogens, such as infantile dyspepsia, frightened, and disharmony of *yin* and *yang*. It is characterized as long term disease, diverse heat tendencies and belongs to deficiency syndrome. Besides, factors of external contraction and internal injury interact.

辨证施治

针对引起发热的病因处理，是对发热处理的关键，只有这样才能从根本上解决发热。因此，对于外感发热的辨证治疗与感冒相同，在此仅谈内伤发热的治疗。

1. 伤食发热

发热以夜暮为甚，腹壁、手心发热，两颧红，口赤，夜卧不安，纳呆，嗳腐吞酸，胸腹胀满，疼痛拒按，便秘或泻下酸臭，唇红，苔白腻或黄腻。

辨证要点　以低热为主，常见手足心热，大便秘结，夜卧不安，纳呆，舌苔黄腻。

治则　消食导滞清热。

取穴　退六腑　清大肠　清胃（图4-1～图4-3）

方义　退六腑为清脏腑郁热以退热；清大肠为清理肠腑以消积除热；清胃经意在泻胃火以消食积。

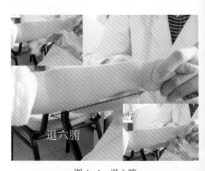

图4-1　退六腑
Picture 4-1　Clearing manipulation on six-*fu* point

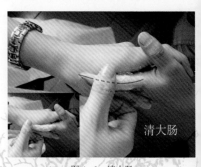

图4-2　清大肠
Picture 4-2　Clearing manipulation on large-intestine-meridian point

Treatment according to syndrome differentiation

The key to resolve fever is to finalise the cause of fever. In this part, we only talk about the treatment for fever of internal injury, because treatment for fever of external contraction is much the same as that of common cold, which will be introduced later.

1 Dyspeptic fever

This fever is characterized as fever aggravated at dust, feverish sensation in abdomen, palms, mouth and cheeks, restless sleep, anorexia, belching, acid regurgitation, stuffiness and fullness in chest and abdomen, pain aggravated by pressing, constipation or stinking diarrhea, red lips, whitish greasy or yellow greasy fur.

- Differentiation guidelines: low fever as main symptom, feverish sensation in palms and soles, constipation, restless sleep, anorexia, and yellow and greasy fur as commonly seen symptoms.

- Therapeutic principle: promoting digestion, removing food stagnation and clearing heat.

- Treatment: clearing manipulation on six-*fu* point, large-intestine-meridian point, and stomach-meridian point. (Picture 4-1 to Picture 4-3)

- Prescription analysis: clearing six-*fu* point means clearing stagnated heat in the viscera to defervesce; clearing large-intestine-meridian point means clearing the large intestine to eliminate the accumulated heat; clearing stomach-meridian point means clearing the stomach fire to eliminate food accumulation.

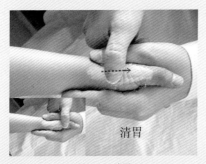

图 4-3 清胃
Picture 4-3 Clearing manipulation on stomach-
meridian point

2. 惊恐发热

发热不甚，昼轻夜重，伴有面色青黄，心悸，睡梦虚惊，甚则睡卧中手足挛缩，骤然啼哭，舌红，苔黄或黄腻。

辨证要点　低热，昼轻夜重，睡梦虚惊，骤然啼哭，舌红苔黄。

治则　平肝清热，镇惊安神。

取穴　平肝　清天河水 捣小天心（图4-4～图4-6）

方义　平肝经意在平肝息风镇静；清天河水为清心泻火以除烦热；捣小天心为镇惊安神。

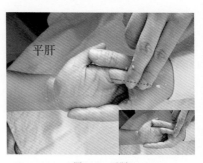

图4-4　平肝
Picture 4-4　Clearing manipulation on liver-meridian point

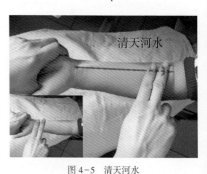

图4-5　清天河水
Picture 4-5　Clearing manipulation on heaven-river-water point

3. 阴虚发热

午后发热，五心烦热，两颧潮红，盗汗，咽干，身体消瘦，口唇干燥，舌红，苔少或无苔。

辨证要点　午后发热，五心烦热，盗汗，舌红，苔少或无苔。

治则　养阴清热。

取穴　运八卦　清天河水 揉二马（图4-7～图4-9）

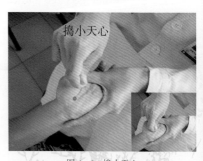

图4-6　捣小天心
Picture 4-6　Pounding small-heaven-center point

方义　运八卦意在健脾和胃，调和气血阴阳；清天河水为清热泻火以除烦，具有清热而不伤阴之功效；揉二马具有滋补阴液、壮水制火之功效，配清天河水具有养阴清热的作用。

2　Frightened fever

This fever is characterized as low fever, fever aggravated in the evening and relieved in the morning, greenish yellow complexion, palpitation, intermittent sleep awakened in fright by nightmare, and even convulsant limbs in sleep, abrupt night crying, red tongue, yellow or yellow and greasy fur.

- Differentiation guidelines: low fever, fever aggravated in the evening, intermittent sleep awakened in fright by nightmare, abrupt night crying, red tongue and yellow fur.
- Therapeutic principle: soothing liver, clearing heat, and inducing sedation and tranquilization.
- Treatment: clearing manipulation on liver-meridian point and heaven-river-water point, and pounding small-heaven-center point. (Picture 4－4 to Picture 4－6)
- Prescription analysis: clearing manipulation on liver-meridian point aims to calm the liver wind and be quiet; clearing manipulation on heaven-river-water point aims to clear heart-fire to eliminate vexation; pounding small-heaven-center point aims to calm fright and tranquilize mind.

3　*Yin*-deficiency fever

This fever is characterized as afternoon fever, vexing heat in chest, palms and soles, tidal fever in cheeks, night sweat, dry throat, mouth and lips, emaciation, red tongue, scarce or no fur.

- Differentiation guidelines: afternoon fever, vexing heat in chest, palms and soles, night sweat, red tongue, scarce or no fur.
- Therapeutic principle: nourishing *yin* and clearing heat.
- Treatment: arc-pushing *bagua* point, clearing manipulation on heaven-river-water point and kneading *erma* point. (Picture 4－7 to Picture 4－9)
- Prescription analysis: arc-pushing *bagua* point aims to strengthen the spleen and stomach, regulate *qi*, blood, *yin* and *yang*; clearing manipulation on heaven-

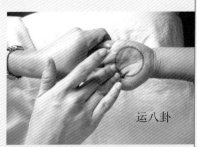

图 4－7　运八卦

Picture 4－7　Arc-pushing *bagua* point

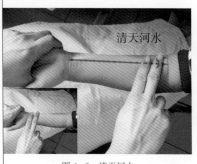

清天河水

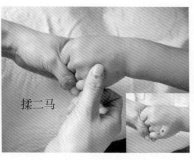

揉二马

图 4-8　清天河水
Picture 4-8　Clearing manipulation on heaven-
　　　　　　　river-water point

图 4-9　揉二马
Picture 4-9　Kneading *erma* point

预防与护理

（1）**加强小儿的护理**　乳贵有时，食贵有节，合理饮食，避免损伤脾胃，造成蕴湿成热。

（2）**增加户外活动**　平日宜适当增加室外活动，以增强机体抵抗力，在传染病流行季节，不到公共场所活动，以免感受时行疫疠之邪。

（3）**避免惊恐外扰**　注意小儿不宜接触异常之物，不要恐吓小儿，不要让小儿看恐怖电视，以免惊恐外扰。

（4）**病后调养**　凡大病之后，必须注意饮食营养与药物调理，以免内伤津液，气血亏损。

（5）**高热患儿的护理**　应注意休息，饮食以清淡为宜；多饮水，以防耗伤津液；服解表发汗之药，应进热饮，如米粥，并盖衣被，以助汗出，但取微汗为宜，不可过汗。

river-water point aims to clear heart-fire to eliminate vexation without injuring *yin*; kneading *erma* point is of the function of restricting *yang* through nourishing *yin*, or nourishing *yin* and clearing heat with clearing heaven-river-water point together.

Prevention and Care

1 Enhanced care: Timing, light diet will avoid spleen and stomach injury which leads to heat transformation from the accumulated dampness.

2 More outdoor activities: Appropriate outdoor activities can enhance the body resistance. In epidemic season of infectious diseases, less activity in public places is recommended to avoid the infection of evil pestilence

3 Avoid terror and fright: Do not let children contact the abnormal things. Do not intimidate children. Do not let children watch horror television programs.

4 Recuperate: After illness, attention must be paid to diet and drug treatment in order to avoid internal injury of the thin and thick fluids causing deficient *qi* and blood.

5 Care for the baby with high fever: Let the baby take a proper rest and light food and drink more water. After taking the sweat-inducing medicine, such measures as taking hot drinks like congee and covering quilt should be taken to help light sweat. Heavy sweat is forbidden.

第二节　感冒

感冒是儿科最常见的外感疾病。一年四季均可发生，冬春两季及气候变化时发病率较高，临床表现为发热、头痛、鼻塞流涕、喷嚏、咳嗽、全身不适。小儿感冒常见夹痰、夹滞、夹惊等兼症。

病因病机

小儿脏腑娇嫩，肌肤疏薄，卫外不固；寒暖不能自调，易于感受外邪。此外，小儿为纯阳之体，肺经平素易有痰热伏火，肺卫失于调节，亦易感外邪。

六淫邪气侵袭人体，以风邪为主因，在不同季节与当令之时气相合而伤人，如：冬季多属风寒，春季多属风热，秋季多兼燥气，梅雨季节多夹湿邪。若四时六气失常，非时之气夹时行病毒伤人，发病不限于季节性，病情重，往往互为传染流行。

肺脏受邪，失于清肃，气机不利，津液凝聚为痰，故感冒易夹痰。

小儿脾常不足，感受风邪，往往影响运化功能，稍有饮食不节，则致乳食停滞不化，阻滞中焦，此为感冒夹滞。

小儿神气怯弱，感邪之后，易心神不宁，出现一时性惊厥，此为感冒夹惊。

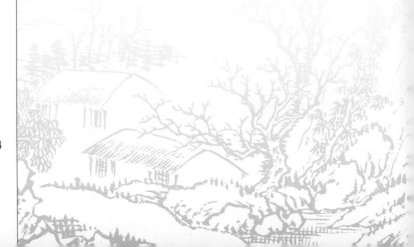

Section 2   Common Cold

Common cold is the most common disease of external contraction in pediatrics. It occurs at any time, but much more often in spring, winter and when climate changes. It manifests as fever, headache, a stuffy and runny nose, sneeze, cough and general malaise. Infantile common cold is usually concurrent with phlegm, stagnation and fright.

Cause and mechanism of disease

Infant has tender viscera, thin skin, insecurity of defensive *qi*, fragile regulation of warm and cold, and thus he/she tends to be invaded by external pathogens. Moreover, infantile constitution is purely *yang*, which is easy to have phlegm-heat congestion in lung meridian, a cause that the defensive *qi* fails to regulate and also is apt to be invaded by external pathogens.

In six excesses, wind-evil is much more common in invading human body. It always combines with seasonal pathogens, for example, wind-cold in winter, wind-heat in spring, wind-dry in autumn, and wind-damp in rainy seasons. And in abnormal seasons, if there are epidemic pathogens, this disease will be serious, contagious and occur in any season.

When the lung catches disease, it fails to purify and *qi* movement becomes disturbed, then fluid is concentrated to phlegm. So, common cold is usually concurrent with phlegm.

Infantile spleen is always insufficient, which when the wind-evil invades, the transportation and transformation functions of the spleen are disturbed and in combination with improper diet, the milk and food remain undigested and stagnate in the middle *jiao*. So, common cold is usually concurrent with stagnation.

Infantile mental activity is frail. It is easy to be disturbed and even temporary syncope will occur when pathogens invade. It is common cold with fright.

辨证施治

1. 风寒感冒

恶寒重，发热轻，无汗，头痛，肢节酸痛，鼻塞声重，时流清涕，喉痒，咳嗽，痰稀薄色白，口不渴或渴喜热饮，舌淡苔薄白而润。

辨证要点 有外感风寒的病史，恶寒重发热轻，无汗，流清涕，口不渴或渴喜热饮。

治则 解表祛风寒。

取穴 揉一窝风 平肝清肺（图4-10、图4-11）

不得汗加拿列缺或加提捏大椎穴；头痛加揉阳池；

鼻塞不通加揉迎香；腹痛加揉外劳宫；

呕吐加清胃。

方义 揉一窝风可通经

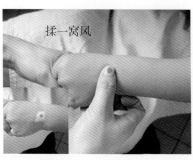

揉一窝风

图4-10 揉一窝风
Picture 4-10　Kneading *yiwofeng* point

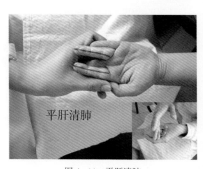

平肝清肺

图4-11 平肝清肺
Picture 4-11　Clearing manipulation on liver-meridian point and lung-meridian point

络、解肌表，可奏发汗祛邪之功；清肝经行气解郁，以防肝火旺盛；清肺经有疏风解表、化痰止咳的作用。对不得汗者，拿列缺或提捏大椎为宣肺散寒之要穴，汗出邪从表解而病愈。此手法宜重，疗效方佳。

2. 风热感冒

身热较著，微恶风，汗泄不畅，头胀痛，咳嗽，痰黏而黄，咽干，或咽喉乳蛾红肿疼痛，鼻塞流黄浊涕，口渴欲饮，舌边尖红苔薄白微黄。

辨证要点 身热恶风，涕浊痰黄，咽红肿痛，口渴欲饮，舌边尖红苔薄黄。

治则 解表邪，祛风热。

Treatment according to syndrome differentiation

1 Wind-cold common cold

This common cold is characterized as serious aversion to cold, low fever, no sweat, headache, aching joints of limbs, a stuffy nose, low voice in speaking, watery nasal discharge, a scratching throat, cough, thin and whitish phlegm, not thirsty or in favor of hot drinking, pale-red tongue, thin, white and moist fur.

• Differentiation guidelines: a medical history of catching external wind-cold pathogen, serious aversion to cold, low fever, no sweat, clear nasal discharge, not thirsty or in favor of hot drinking.

• Therapeutic principle: releasing exterior and dispelling wind-cold.

• Treatment: kneading *yiwofeng* point, clearing manipulation on liver-meridian point and lung-meridian point. (Picture 4 – 10, Picture 4 – 11)

If sweat is still not induced after mentioned-above manipulations, add pinching point of *Dazhui* (GV 14) or grasping point of *lieque* ; add kneading *yangchi* point for headache; add kneading *Yingxiang* (LI 20) point for a stuffy nose; add kneading dorsal-*laogong* point for abdominal pain; add clearing manipulation on stomach-meridian point for vomiting.

• Prescription analysis: kneading *yiwofeng* point can dredge meridians and release the fleshy exterior with the function of inducing sweating to eliminate pathogen; clearing manipulation on liver-meridian point can promote *qi* circulation and remove stagnation to prevent excessive liver-fire; clearing manipulation on lung-meridian point has the function of dispersing wind to release exterior, and eliminating phlegm to stop cough. Grasping *lieque* point or *Dazhui* (GV14) is good at ventilating the lung and dispersing cold and therefore is suitable for the patient without sweating. Heavy manipulation gives rise to a good effect.

2 Wind-heat common cold

This common cold is characterized as high fever, slightly aversion to wind, difficult sweating, distending pain in head, cough, yellow and sticky phlegm, dry throat or red and sore tonsil, a stuffy nose, yellow and turbid nasal discharge, thirsty and in favor of drinking, redness in the edge and tip of tongue, thin, white and yellowish fur.

• Differentiation guidelines: high fever, aversion to wind, turbid nasal discharge, yellow phlegm, red and sore throat, redness in the edge and tip of

77

取穴　平肝　清肺　清天河水（图4-12～图4-14）

头痛加揉阳池；鼻塞不通加黄蜂入洞；

腹泻加清补大肠、清补脾；高热者将清天河水改为退六腑。

方义　清肝经以行气解郁，清肺经以宣肺清热，疏风解表；清天河水有清热解表的作用。

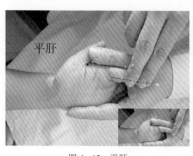

图4-12　平肝
Picture 4-12　Clearing manipulation on liver-meridian point

3. 兼证

（1）挟痰　兼见咳嗽较剧，咳声重浊，喉中痰鸣，舌苔厚腻。

辨证要点　肺卫表证伴咳嗽痰多，以风热为主。

治则　解表祛风热，兼宽胸理气化痰。

取穴　平肝清肺　清天河水　运八卦（图4-15～图4-17）

痰盛者加清补脾；高热者将清天河水改为退六腑。

方义　小儿为纯阳之体，感邪后易从热化，故兼证的治疗均在风热感冒的基础上加穴治疗。夹痰者在平肝清肺、清天河水的基础上，加顺运八卦以宽胸利膈，理气化痰；痰湿壅盛者清补脾经以达健脾助运之功；热盛者退六腑以清腑泄

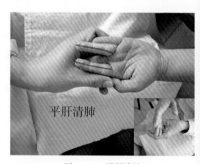

图4-15　平肝清肺
Picture 4-15　Clearing manipulation on liver-meridian point and lung-meridian point

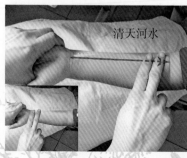

图4-16　清天河水
Picture 4-16　Clearing manipulation on heaven-river-water point

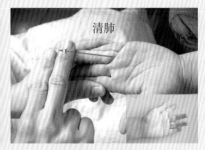

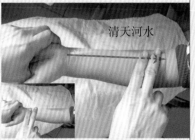

图 4-13 清肺
Picture 4-13 Clearing manipulation on lung-
meridian point

图 4-14 清天河水
Picture 4-14 Clearing manipulation
on heaven-river-water point

tongue, thin and yellowish fur.

● Therapeutic principle: releasing exterior, repelling wind-heat.

● Treatment: clearing manipulation on liver-meridian point, lung-meridian point and heaven-river-water point. (Picture 4-12 to Picture 4-14)

Add kneading *yangchi* point for headache; add manipulation called *huangfengrudong* for a stuffy nose; add pushing large-intestine-meridian point and spleen-meridian point to and fro for diarrhea; add pushing six-*fu* point for persistent high fever.

● Prescription analysis: clearing manipulation on liver-meridian point aims to promote *qi* circulation and remove stagnation; clearing manipulation on lung-meridian point aims to ventilate the lung to clear heat, and disperse wind to release exterior; clearing manipulation on heaven-river-water point has the function of clearing heat and releasing exterior.

3 Complications

a. Concurrent with phlegm: accompanied by more serious cough with deep and harsh sound, lots of phlegm in throat and sounding with respiration, thick and greasy fur.

● Differentiation guidelines: defensive exterior syndrome involving lung system, together with cough and lots of phlegm. It is chiefly caused by wind-heat pathogen.

● Therapeutic principle: releasing exterior, repelling wind-heat, soothing chest, regulating *qi* and resolving phlegm.

● Treatment: clearing manipulation on liver-meridian point, lung-meridian point and heaven-river-water point, and arc-pushing *bagua* point.

79

热，使邪有出处。

（2）**挟滞** 兼见脘腹胀满，不思饮食，呕吐酸腐，口气秽浊，大便酸臭，或腹痛泄泻，或大便秘结，小便短赤，舌苔厚腻。

辨证要点 肺卫表证加腹胀、纳差等不消化症状。

治则 解表祛风热，兼理气化积。

取穴 平肝清肺 清天河水 运八卦 清补脾（图4-15～图4-18）

呕吐加清胃；高热者将清天河水改为退六腑。

方义 夹滞者在平肝清肺、清天河水的基础上，加顺运八卦以理气消食化积；清补脾经可运脾健胃以消积滞。高热者退六腑以清腑泄热，使邪有出处。

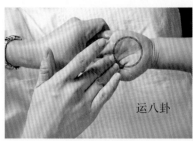

运八卦

图4-17 运八卦
Picture 4-17 Arc-pushing *bagua* point

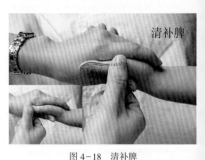

清补脾

图4-18 清补脾
Picture 4-18 Pushing spleen-meridian point to and fro

（3）**挟惊** 兼见惊惕啼叫，睡卧不安，甚至出现惊厥，舌尖红。

辨证要点 肺卫表证伴躁动不安，惊惕啼叫。

治则 解表祛风热，安神镇惊。

取穴 平肝（加重）清肺 清天河水（加重）捣小天心（图4-19～图4-22）

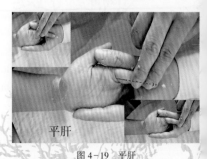

平肝

图4-19 平肝
Picture 4-19 Clearing manipulation on liver-meridian point

(Picture 4 – 15 to Picture 4 – 17)

Add pushing spleen-meridian point to and fro for phlegm in a large mount; add pushing six-*fu* point instead of clearing heaven-river-water point for high fever.

- Prescription analysis: Infantile constitution is purely *yang*, which is easy to become heat symptom after pathogen infection, so some point/ points is/are added to treat complications based on wind-heat common cold. Concurrent with phlegm: add arc-pushing *bagua* point to free chest and diaphragm, regulate *qi*-flowing to eliminate phlegm; pushing spleen-meridian point to and fro to eliminate phlegm in a large mount has the function of invigorating the spleen to aid in transportation; add pushing six-*fu* point aims to let the heat out of *fu*-organs with defecation.

b. Concurrent with stagnation: together with stuffiness and fullness in stomach and abdomen, no appetite, acid and putrid vomiting, smelly mouth, stinking stool or painful diarrhea or constipation, dark and short-flow urine, thick and greasy fur.

- Differentiation guidelines: defensive exterior syndrome involving lung system, together with symptoms of dyspepsia, such as abdominal distension and anorexia.
- Therapeutic principle: releasing exterior, repelling wind-heat, regulating *qi* movement and resolving stagnation.
- Treatment: clearing manipulation on liver-meridian point, lung-meridian point, and heaven-river-water point, and arc-pushing *bagua* point, and pushing spleen-meridian point to and fro. (Picture 4 – 15 to Picture 4 – 18)

Add clearing stomach-meridian point for vomiting; add pushing six-*fu* point instead of clearing heaven-river-water point for high fever.

- Prescription analysis: add arc-pushing *bagua* point to regulate *qi*-flowing, promote digestion, and remove food stagnation; add pushing spleen-meridian point to and fro to strengthen the spleen and stomach to remove food stagnation; pushing six-*fu* point is added for high fever to clear the *fu*-organ to discharge heat.

c. Concurrent with fright: together with scream due to fright, restless sleep, and even frightened syncope, red tongue tip.

- Differentiation guidelines: defensive exterior syndrome involving

81

高热者将清天河水改为退六腑。

方义 小儿神气怯弱，肝常有余，感邪后易心神不宁，烦躁不安，故重用清肝经以镇惊安神，平肝息风；与清天河水并重加强清热泻火之功；清肺经以宣肺清热解表；捣小天心以加强清心安神之功。

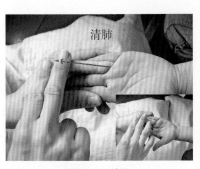

图4-20 清肺
Picture 4-20 Clearing manipulation on lung-meridian point

预防与护理

（1）**积极锻炼** 利用自然因素锻炼身体十分重要，户外活动和体育锻炼，都是积极的方法，要持之以恒，经常进行，就能增强体质，防止感冒。

（2）**讲卫生，避免发病诱因** 衣服穿得过多或过少，室温过高或过低，天气骤变，环境污染和被动吸烟等，都是感冒的诱因。

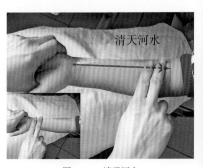

图4-21 清天河水
Picture 4-21 Clearing manipulation on heaven-river-water point

（3）**避免交叉感染** 在家庭中成人患者避免与健康儿接触，且要注意室内通风。

（4）**饮食宜忌** 患病期间应多喝开水，多食新鲜水果、蔬菜。饮食宜清淡，避免肥甘厚味影响脾胃运化吸收。

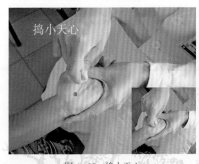

图4-22 捣小天心
Picture 4-22 Pounding small-heaven-center point

（5）**发热患儿要注意控制体温** 避免体温突然上升引起惊厥。

lung system, together with restlessness, scream due to fright.

• Therapeutic principle: releasing exterior, repelling wind-heat, and inducing sedation and tranquilization.

• Treatment: clearing manipulation on liver-meridian point, lung-meridian point and heaven-river-water point for longer duration, and pounding small-heaven-center point. (Picture 4 – 19 to Picture 4 – 22)

Add pushing six-*fu* point instead of clearing heaven-river-water point for high fever.

• Prescription analysis: Infantile mental activity is frail and his/her liver is often in superabundance. It is easy to be disturbed and marked by dysphoria and therefore clearing manipulation on liver-meridian point for longer time is added to calm fright, tranquilize mind and liver wind; strengthen the power of clearing heat with clearing heaven-river-water point; clearing manipulation on lung-meridian point aims to ventilate the lung, clear heat and release exterior; pounding small-heaven-center point aims to strengthen the power of clearing away the heart fire and tranquilizing mind.

Prevention and Care

1 Active exercise: It is very important to do physical exercise under natural factors. Both outdoor activities and exercises are positive approaches. Keep practicing regularly will invigorate health effectively and prevent a cold.

2 Paying attention to hygiene and avoid predisposing factors: Common cold can be induced by such predisposing factors as wearing too many or too few clothes, too high or too low room temperature, sudden change of the weather, environmental pollution, passive smoking and so on.

3 Avoid cross infection: Adult patients should avoid contact with healthy children at home, and pay attention to the indoor ventilation.

4 Proper diet and food prohibition: Stick to a light diet and avoid fat and rich food affecting the absorption of the spleen and stomach. Drink enough warm boiled water, and eat more fresh fruit and vegetables during the illness.

5 Paying attention to body temperature control for baby with fever: Avoid infantile convulsion due to sudden rise of the body temperature.

83

第三节　咳嗽

咳嗽是小儿呼吸系统最常见的症状，是由于呼吸道炎症、异物或其他物理、化学因素刺激呼吸道黏膜，通过咳嗽中枢引起的咳嗽动作。咳嗽是一种保护性反射，通过咳嗽可将呼吸道异物或分泌物排除体外。

病因病机

小儿形气未充，卫外功能较差，易感外邪，使肺失宣降；肺气上逆则发为咳嗽；小儿脾胃薄弱，乳食生冷所伤致脾失健运，痰浊内生，而上贮于肺，肺失宣肃，发生咳嗽。另外，小儿禀赋不足，肺脾气虚，则易致肺气耗伤或肺脾气虚之咳嗽。小儿咳嗽的致病因素虽多，但发病机制则一，皆须肺脏受累才能发生。

辨证施治

1. 风寒咳嗽

咳嗽频作，喉痒严重，痰稀色白，鼻塞流涕，恶寒无汗，发热头痛，舌苔薄白。

辨证要点　咳嗽声重，咳痰稀白，伴有风寒表证。

治则　解表祛风寒，宣肺理气。

取穴　运八卦　平肝　清肺　推四横纹（图4-23～图4-25）

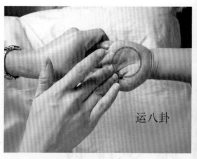

运八卦

图4-23　运八卦
Picture 4-23　Arc-pushing *bagua* point

方义　顺运八卦能宽胸顺气而化痰；清肝经行气化痰而止咳；清肺经解表宣肺，化痰止咳；推四横纹宽胸理气，化痰止咳。

Section 3   Cough

Cough is the pediatric respiratory movement reflected through the cough nerve center by various factors stimulating mucous membrane of respiratory tract. The factors are respiratory inflammation, foreign substance or other physical and chemical factors. It is the most common symptom in respiratory system of pediatrics. It is a protective reflection and through which, the foreign substance and secretion in respiratory tract are drained away.

Cause and mechanism of disease

Infant is immature. Due to insecurity of defensive function, infant tends to catch exterior pathogens and the lung fails to purify and ventilate. Wherever there is adverse rising of lung qi, there is cough. Moreover, infantile spleen and stomach are tender. If raw and cold milk or food impairs them, the spleen fails to transport, and phlegm-turbidity is engendered interior, which is deposited in the lung. Then the lung fails to purify and ventilate, inducing cough. In addition, infantile innate endowment is insufficient and lung and spleen qi are deficient, so infantile cough usually has syndrome of lung impairment or lung and spleen qi deficiency. Though causes of infantile cough are diverse, the only single mechanism is the function of lung is affected.

Treatment according to syndrome differentiation

1   Wind-cold cough

This cough is characterized as frequent cough, terribly scratching throat, thin and whitish phlegm, a stuffy nose, nasal discharge, aversion to cold, no sweat, fever, headache, thin and white fur.

• Differentiation guidelines: cough, low voice in speaking, thin and whitish phlegm, accompanied with wind-cold exterior syndrome.

• Therapeutic principle: releasing exterior and repelling wind-cold, ventilating lung and regulating qi.

• Treatment: arc-pushing $bagua$, clearing liver-meridian point and lung-meridian point, and pushing four-transverse-crease point. (Picture 4-23 to Picture 4-25)

• Prescription analysis: arc-pushing $bagua$ clockwise can free chest, smooth qi flow and clear phlegm; clearing liver-meridian point

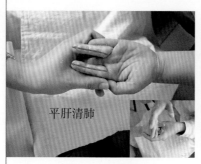

平肝清肺

图 4-24 平肝清肺
Picture 4-24 Clearing manipulation on liver-
meridian point and lung-meridian point

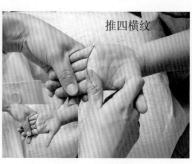

推四横纹

图 4-25 推四横纹
Picture 4-25 Pushing four-transverse-crease
point

2. 风热咳嗽

咳嗽不爽，痰黄黏稠，不易咳出，咽痛口渴，鼻流浊涕，伴有发热头痛，恶风，微汗出，舌苔薄黄。

辨证要点 咳嗽频剧，咳痰黄稠，咽痛，伴有风热表证。

治则 解表祛风热，清肺止咳。

取穴 运八卦 平肝清肺 清胃 退六腑（图 4-23、图 4-24、图 4-26、图 4-27）

方义 顺运八卦能宽胸顺气而化痰；清肝经、清肺经宣肺清热，化痰止咳；清胃经清胃降逆，利咽止咳；退六腑清热通腑以除热痰。

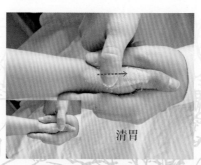

清胃

图 4-26 清胃
Picture 4-26 Clearing manipulation on stomach-
meridian point

can promote *qi* flow and eliminate phlegm to relieve cough; clearing lung-meridian point is able to release exterior and ventilate the lung, and eliminate phlegm to relieve cough; pushing four-transverse-crease point is able to free chest and regulate *qi* flow and eliminate phlegm to relieve cough.

2 Wind-heat cough

This cough is characterized as cough, sticky and yellow phlegm, difficulty in coughing up, sore throat, thirsty, turbid nasal discharge, fever, headache, aversion to wind, slightly sweating, thin and yellowish fur.

- Differentiation guidelines: serious and frequent cough, sticky and yellow phlegm, sore throat, accompanied with wind-heat exterior syndrome.

- Therapeutic principle: releasing exterior and repelling wind-heat, clearing lung and relieving cough

- Treatment: arc-pushing *bagua* point, clearing manipulation on liver-meridian point, lung-meridian point, stomach-meridian point, and six-*fu* point. (Picture 4 – 23, Picture 4 – 24, Picture 4 – 26, Picture 4 – 27)

- Prescription analysis: arc-pushing *bagua* point clockwise can free chest and regulate *qi* flow to eliminate phlegm; clearing liver-meridian point and lung-meridian point are able to ventilate lung and clear heat, and eliminate phlegm to relieve cough; clearing stomach-meridian point is able to clear the stomach to ascend *qi* flow, and relieve sore throat and cough; clearing six-*fu* point is able to purge six-*fu* to eliminate heat and phlegm.

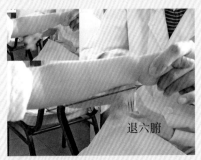

图 4 – 27　退六腑
Picture 4 – 27　Clearing manipulation on six-*fu*
point

3. 痰湿咳嗽

咳嗽反复发作，咳声重浊，因痰而咳，痰出咳平，每遇早晨或食后则咳甚，食少，体倦，大便时溏，舌苔白腻。

辨证要点 咳声重浊，反复发作，每遇清晨或食后加重，多伴有脾虚证。

治则 益气降逆，培土生金。

取穴 清肺 清补脾 运八卦（图4-28～图4-30）

方义 清肺经宣肺化痰止咳；清补脾经意在运脾化湿，脾能健运，痰湿渐化，则咳嗽可愈；顺运八卦以宽胸理气，化痰止咳。

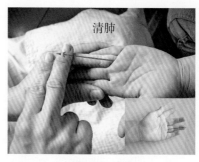

清肺

图4-28 清肺
Picture 4-28 Clearing manipulation on lung-meridian point

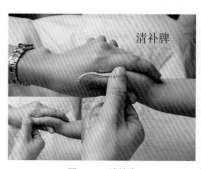

清补脾

图4-29 清补脾
Picture 4-29 Pushing spleen-meridian point to and fro

4. 阴虚咳嗽

干咳，咳声短促，痰少黏白，口干咽燥，手足心热，夜寐盗汗，舌红少苔。

辨证要点 干咳少痰伴有肺阴虚证。

治则 益气降逆，滋阴润燥。

取穴 清肺（加重） 清补脾 揉二马（图4-31～图4-33）

方义 清肺经意在宣肺化痰止咳，加重推拿手法以清其余热；清补脾以健脾益肺；揉二马以养阴生津，使阴液充沛则燥咳自止。

3　Phlegm-dampness cough

This cough is characterized as repeated occurrence of cough with deep and harsh sound, cough induced by phlegm and relieved by spitting the phlegm, cough aggravated in the morning and after eating, no appetite, lassitude, occasional loose stool, greasy and whitish fur.

- Differentiation guidelines: repeated occurrence of cough with deep and harsh sound, cough aggravated in the morning and after eating, often accompanied with spleen deficiency syndrome.

- Therapeutic principle: invigorating *qi* and checking adverse rising of *qi*, nourishing spleen to benefit lung.

- Treatment: clearing manipulation on lung-meridian point, pushing spleen-meridian point to and fro, arc-pushing *bagua* point. (Picture 4−28 to Picture 4−30)

- Prescription analysis: clearing manipulation on lung-meridian point can ventilate the lung, eliminate phlegm to relieve cough; pushing spleen-meridian point to and fro can activate the spleen to eliminate dampness and phlegm and relieve cough; arc-pushing *bagua* point clockwise is able to free chest, regulate *qi* flow, eliminate phlegm to relieve cough.

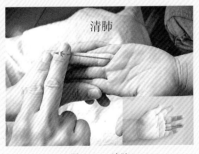

图 4−30　运八卦
Picture 4−30　Arc-pushing *bagua* point

4　*Yin*-deficiency cough

This cough is characterized as dry and brief cough, sticky and whitish phlegm in small amounts, dry mouth and throat, feverish sensation in palms and soles, night sweat, red tongue and scarce fur.

- Differentiation guidelines: dry cough, small amounts of phlegm, accompanied with lung *yin* deficiency syndrome.

- Therapeutic principle: invigorating *qi* and checking adverse rising

图 4−31　清肺
Picture 4−31　Clearing manipulation on lung-meridian point

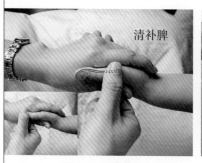

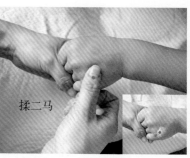

图 4-32　清补脾
Picture 4-32　Pushing spleen-meridian point to and fro

图 4-33　揉二马
Picture 4-33　Kneading *erma* point

5．肺虚久咳

咳而无力，痰白清稀，面色㿠白，气短懒言，动则汗出，食少便溏，舌淡。

辨证要点　肺虚与脾虚并见。

治则　滋阴润燥，培土生金。

取穴　揉二马　清补脾（图 4-33、图 4-32）

方义　肺金在上宜清肃，肾水在下宜上滋，金水相生，揉二马以滋阴润肺，顺气化痰而除久咳；清补脾经以健脾助运，达培土生金之功。

预防与护理

（1）**加强锻炼，防止感冒**　小儿咳嗽以外感居多，而外感咳嗽又以感受风邪为多，因而在日常生活中，应注意增加孩子的户外活动，加强运动锻炼，增强体质，减少感冒的次数，同时，衣着要适宜，避免外邪入内而致咳嗽。

（2）**合理饮食，顾护脾胃**　小儿咳嗽虽然以外感风邪为多，但内伤饮食咳嗽者亦不少见，因而在饮食喂养中，少吃辛辣香燥食物，生冷饮料应当戒，肥甘厚味不宜过度，以免饮食内伤脾胃而滋生痰液。

（3）**明确诊断，避免误诊**　对于反复咳嗽的患儿应注意清理鼻咽部的慢性病灶，明确病因，避免误诊而延误病情。

of *qi*, nourishing *yin* and moistening dryness.

• Treatment: clearing manipulation on lung-meridian point for longer duration, pushing spleen-meridian point to and fro, kneading *erma* point. (Picture 4−31 to Picture 4−33)

• Prescription analysis: clearing manipulation on lung-meridian point is able to ventilate the lung, eliminate phlegm to relieve cough, the longer duration is able to clear heat more effectively; pushing spleen-meridian point to and fro is able to tonify the spleen and lung; kneading *erma* point can nourish *yin* and produce thin fluid and abundant *yin* fluids make dry cough cease.

5 Chronic lung deficiency cough

This cough is characterized as cough lack of strength, watery and whitish phlegm, pale complexion, short breath, reluctant to speak, easy to sweat even after a slight movement, no appetite, loose stool, pale tongue.

• Differentiation guidelines: both of lung deficiency and spleen deficiency syndromes.

• Therapeutic principle: nourishing *yin* and moistening dryness, nourishing spleen to benefit lung.

• Treatment: kneading *erma* point, pushing spleen-meridian point to and fro. (Picture 4−33; Picture 4−32)

• Prescription analysis: lung gold locates on the upper part, it needs clearing, kidney water locates on the lower part, it needs nourishing, gold and water generate with each other. Kneading *erma* is able to nourish *yin* and lung, smooth *qi* flow, and eliminate phlegm to relieve chronic cough. Pushing spleen-meridian point to and fro can activate the spleen to promote transportation and therefore bank up earth to generate metal.

Prevention and Care

1 Active exercise and avoiding cold: Infantile cough is mainly caused by exogenous pathogenic factors, especially by pathogenic wind mostly. So a baby needs more outdoor activities and active exercise in daily life. Reduce the number of colds by way of enhancing physical fitness. At the same time, parents should clothe their children fitly to avoid cough due to internal invasion of the exogenous pathogenic factors.

2 Proper diet and care for the spleen and stomach: Endogenous cough is not rarely seen yet, while exogenous cough is in the majority for

第四节 呕吐

呕吐是食管、胃肠道内容物经口腔吐出，呕吐时食管、胃或肠道呈逆蠕动，伴有腹肌、膈肌强烈收缩。恶心是一种可以引起呕吐冲动的胃内不适感，常是呕吐的先兆。小儿在哺乳后乳汁自口角唇边流出，称为溢乳。多因哺乳过急过多所致，一般不视为病象。

病因病机

中医学认为，胃为"水谷之海"，主受纳腐熟水谷，以降为顺，凡乳食内伤，外感六淫，胃中蕴热或脾胃虚寒，胃阴不足，肝气犯胃，暴受惊恐等可影响胃的正常功能，导致胃失和降而引起呕吐。呕吐的病因各不相同，但其病机总属胃失和降、胃气上逆所致。

辨证施治

1. 伤食呕吐

呕吐酸腐，不思饮食，脘腹胀满，吐后觉舒，大便秘结或泻下，苔厚腻。

辨证要点　多有伤食病史，呕吐酸腐，腹胀，舌苔厚腻。

治则　消积降逆止吐。

取穴　揉板门　运八卦清胃　清补脾（图4-34～图4-37）

方义　揉板门以健脾和胃，消食化积，通调三焦之气；顺运八卦行滞消食，降逆止呕；清胃经具有和胃降

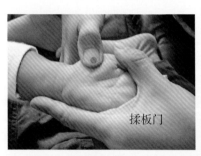

揉板门

图4-34　揉板门
Picture 4-34　Kneading *banmen* point

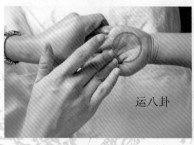

运八卦

图4-35　运八卦
Picture 4-35　Arc-pushing *bagua* point

children. The children need less spicy, fragrant and dry food, less greasy food, and no cold drinks to avoid the production of phlegm due to internal injury of the spleen and stomach by food.

3 Making diagnosis clear and avoiding misdiagnosis: For the children with recurrent cough, pay attention to eliminating the chronic focus in the nasopharynx to avoid misdiagnosis and condition-delaying.

Section 4 Vomiting

Vomiting is the course of throwing up contents from intestine, stomach and esophagus through mouth, accompanied with adverse peristalsis of intestine, stomach and esophagus, and strong contractions of abdominal muscle and diaphragm muscle. Nausea is uneasiness in stomach, which may urge to vomit and more often than not, is an indication of vomiting. Milk regurgitation refers to the outflow of milk from infantile mouth after nursing. It is usually caused by a too fast breast-feeding and is not regarded as a disease.

Cause and mechanism of disease

In TCM, stomach is the sea of food, which governs intake and digestion. Stomach qi is descending. Normal function of stomach will be affected if there are pathogens like internal injury of infantile diet, attacked by six excesses, heat accumulation in stomach, cold-deficiency of spleen and stomach, stomach yin-deficiency, liver qi impairing stomach or a sudden panic. When the stomach qi fails to descend and is in disharmony, there will be vomiting. Though causes of vomiting are diverse, the chief mechanism is the failure of stomach qi to descend and in disharmony, leading to the adverse rising of stomach qi.

Treatment according to syndrome differentiation

1 Dyspeptic vomiting

This vomiting is characterized as throwing up acid and putrid formula, no appetite, distention and fullness of stomach and abdomen, relieved by vomiting, constipation or diarrhea, thick and greasy fur.

• Differentiation guidelines: medical history of dyspepsia, throwing up acid and putrid formula, distending abdomen, thick and greasy fur.

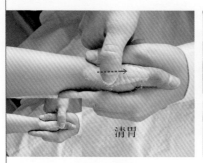

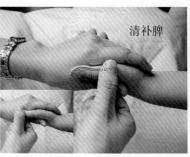

图 4－36　清胃
Picture 4－36　Clearing manipulation on
stomach-meridian point

图 4－37　清补脾
Picture 4－37　Pushing spleen-meridian point
to and fro

逆止呕之功；清补脾经运脾消食化积。

2．胃热呕吐

呕吐频繁，食入即吐，吐物酸臭，口渴多饮，面赤唇红，烦躁少寐，舌红苔黄。

辨证要点　食入即吐，吐物酸臭，口渴多饮，舌红苔黄。

治则　清胃和中降逆。

取穴　清胃　平肝　清天河水　运八卦（图 4－38～图 4－41）

腹痛加揉板门；便秘加清大肠。

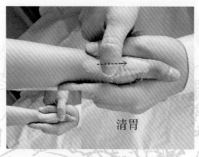

图 4－38　清胃
Picture 4－38　Clearing manipulation on stomach-
meridian point

- Therapeutic principle: removing food stagnation, checking adverse rise of *qi* and stopping vomiting.

- Treatment: kneading *banmen* point, arc-pushing *bagua* point, clearing manipulation on stomach-meridian point, pushing spleen-meridian point to and fro. (Picture 4 – 34 to Picture 4 – 37)

- Prescription analysis: Kneading *banmen* point is able to activate the spleen and harmonize the stomach, resolve stuffiness and food stagnation, harmonize *qi* in the *sanjiao*; arc-pushing *bagua* point clockwise is able to transport stuffiness and food stagnation, descend stomach *qi* to relieve vomiting; clearing manipulation on stomach-meridian point can harmonize the stomach and descend stomach *qi* to stop vomiting; pushing spleen-meridian point to and fro is able to activate the spleen and resolve stuffiness and food stagnation.

2　Stomach-heat vomiting

This vomiting is characterized as frequent occurrence of vomiting soon after eating, throwing up acid and putrid formula, thirsty and in favor of drinking, red complexion and lips, restlessness, insomnia, red tongue and yellow fur.

- Differentiation guidelines: vomiting soon after eating, throwing up acid and putrid formula, thirsty and in favor of drinking, red tongue and yellow fur.

- Therapeutic principle: clearing stomach, harmonizing middle *jiao* and checking adverse rising of *qi*.

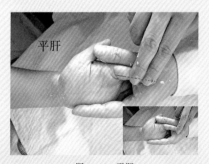

图 4 – 39　平肝
Picture 4 – 39　Clearing manipulation on liver-meridian point

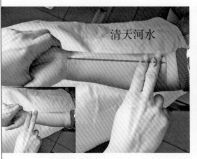

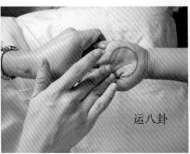

图 4－40　清天河水
Picture 4－40　Clearing manipulation on
heaven-river-water point

图 4－41　运八卦
Picture 4－41　Arc-pushing *bagua* point

方义　清胃经和胃降逆止呕，清肝经疏肝理气和胃，配合清天河水达到清胃泻火之功；顺运八卦以顺气降逆而止呕。

3. 胃寒呕吐

食久方吐，或朝食暮吐，吐出物多为清稀痰水，或不消化乳食残渣，伴面色苍白，精神疲倦，四肢欠温，食少不化，腹痛便溏，唇舌淡白。

辨证要点　朝食暮吐，吐物多为清稀痰水，伴面色苍白，腹痛便溏，舌淡白。

治则　温中降逆止吐。

取穴　揉外劳宫　揉板门　平肝　清胃　运八卦（图 4－42～图 4－46）

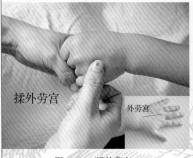

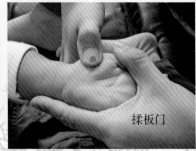

图 4－42　揉外劳宫
Picture 4－42　Kneading dorsal-*laogong* point

图 4－43　揉板门
Picture 4－43　Kneading *banmen* point

- Treatment: clearing manipulation on stomach-meridian point, liver-meridian point, and heaven-river-water point, and arc-pushing *bagua* point. (Picture 4–38 to Picture 4–41)

Add kneading *banmen* point for abdominal pain; add clearing manipulation on large-intestine-meridian point for constipation.

- Prescription analysis: Clearing stomach-meridian point is able to harmonize the stomach and descend stomach *qi* to stop vomiting; clearing liver-meridian point can smooth the liver, regulate *qi*, and harmonize the stomach, clearing heaven-river-water point is combined to clear the stomach and purge fire; arc-pushing *bagua* point clockwise is able to harmonize *qi* to stop vomiting.

3 Stomach-cold vomiting

This vomiting is characterized as vomiting long after eating or morning eating and evening vomiting, throwing up watery phlegm or undigested dregs of milk and food, pale complexion, listlessness, lack of warmth limbs, anorexia, dyspepsia, abdominal pain, loose stool, pale tongue and lips.

- Differentiation guidelines: morning eating and evening vomiting, throwing up watery phlegm, pale complexion, abdominal pain, loose stool, pale tongue and lips.

- Therapeutic principle: warming the middle *jiao*, checking the adverse rising of *qi* and arresting vomiting.

- Treatment: kneading dorsal-*laogong* point and *banmen* point, clearing manipulation on liver-meridian and stomach-meridian point, and

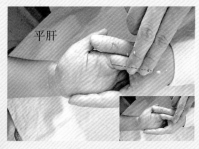
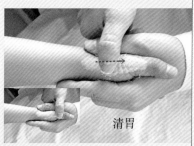

图 4–44　平肝
Picture 4–44　Clearing manipulation on liver-meridian point

图 4–45　清胃
Picture 4–45　Clearing manipulation on stomach-meridian point

方义　揉外劳宫温中散寒；揉板门健脾和胃，通调三焦之气；清肝经疏肝理气和胃；清胃经以和胃降逆止呕；顺运八卦以理气导滞止呕。

4. 胃阴不足呕吐

呕吐反复发作，常呈干呕，饥而不欲进食，口燥，咽干，唇红，大便干结如羊屎，舌红少苔。

辨证要点　呕吐反复发作，干呕，咽干不适，大便干结，舌红少苔。

治则　清补脾胃，降逆止呕。

取穴　揉二马　清胃　运八卦　清补脾（图4-47～图4-50）

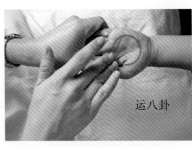

图4-46　运八卦
Picture 4-46　Arc-pushing *bagua* point

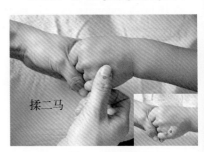

图4-47　揉二马
Picture 4-47　Kneading *erma* point

方义　揉二马养阴生津而润燥；清胃经和胃降逆而止呕；顺运八卦理气导滞，以调和阴阳；清补脾经健脾助运以降胃气。

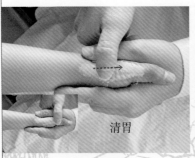

清胃

图4-48　清胃
Picture 4-48　Clearing manipulation on stomach-meridian point

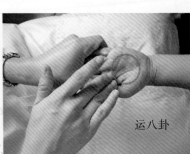

运八卦

图4-49　运八卦
Picture 4-49　Arc-pushing *bagua* point

arc-pushing *bagua* point. (Picture 4 – 42 to Picture 4 – 46)

• Prescription analysis: Kneading dorsal-*laogong* point is able to warm the middle *jiao* and expel cold; kneading *banmen* point is able to activate the spleen and harmonize the stomach and *qi* in the *sanjiao*; clearing liver-meridian point is able to smooth the liver, regulate *qi* and harmonize the stomach; clearing stomach-meridian point is able to harmonize the stomach, descend adverse *qi* to stop vomiting; arc-pushing *bagua* point clockwise is able to harmonize *qi*, dredge indigestion and stop vomiting.

4 Stomach *yin*-deficiency vomiting

This vomiting is characterized as frequent occurrence of vomiting, often retches, hungry but no appetite, dry mouth and throat, red lips, dry and granular stool like sheep excrement, red lips and scarce fur.

• Differentiation guidelines: frequent occurrence of vomiting, often retches, dry throat, dry and granular stool, red lips and scarce fur.

• Therapeutic principle: harmonizing spleen and stomach, checking adverse rising of *qi* and arresting vomiting.

• Treatment: kneading *erma* point, clearing manipulation on stomach-meridian point, arc-pushing *bagua* point, and pushing spleen-meridian point to and fro. (Picture 4 – 47 to Picture 4 – 50)

• Prescription analysis: Kneading *erma* point is able to nourish *yin* and produce thin fluid and moisten dryness; clearing stomach-meridian point is able to harmonize the stomach, descend adverse *qi* to stop vomiting; arc-pushing *bagua*

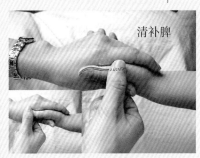

图 4 – 50　清补脾
Picture 4 – 50　Pushing spleen-meridian point to and fro

point clockwise is able to harmonize *qi*, dredge indigestion, harmonize *yin-yang*; pushing spleen-meridian point to and fro is able to activate the spleen and aid in transportation to descend stomach *qi*.

5. 惊恐呕吐

跌仆惊恐后，呕吐清涎，面色忽青忽白，心神烦乱，睡卧不安或惊惕哭闹。

辨证要点 有跌仆惊恐的病史，呕吐清涎，睡卧不安或惊惕哭闹。

治则 平肝镇惊，降逆止呕。

取穴 平肝 清胃 运八卦 清天河水 捣小天心（图4-51～图4-55）

方义 小儿神气怯弱，惊则气乱，肝失疏泄，横逆犯胃，清肝经疏肝镇惊，降逆止呕；清胃经以加强降逆止呕之功效；顺运八卦理气导滞，以调和阴阳；清天河水以清心泻火，除扰心之邪热；捣小天心以镇惊安神。

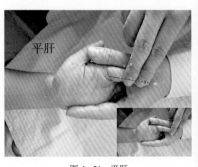

图4-51 平肝
Picture 4-51　Clearing manipulation on liver-meridian point

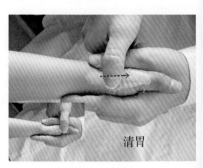

图4-52 清胃
Picture 4-52　Clearing manipulation on stomach-meridian point

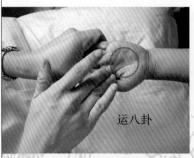

图4-53 运八卦
Picture 4-53　Arc-pushing *bagua* point

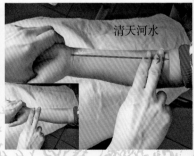

图4-54 清天河水
Picture 4-54　Clearing manipulation on heaven-river-water point

5　Frightened vomiting

This vomiting is characterized as vomiting after falling over and being frightened, throwing up liquid, looming blue of pale complexion, vexing, restless sleep or cry and scream due to fright.

- Differentiation guidelines: medical history of falling over and frightened, throwing up liquid, restless sleep or cry and scream due to fright.

- Therapeutic principle: pacifying liver and inducing tranquilization, checking adverse rising of *qi* and arresting vomiting.

- Treatment: clearing manipulation on liver-meridian point and stomach-meridian point, arc-pushing *bagua* point, clearing manipulation on heaven-river-water point, pounding small-heaven-center point. (Picture 4 – 51 to Picture 4 – 55)

- Prescription analysis: Infants have weak spirit, easily suffered from *qi* disorder due to fright and his/her liver fails to govern the free flow of *qi* and invade the stomach transversely. Clearing manipulation on liver-meridian point is able to relax liver *qi* and relieve convulsion, descend adverse flow of *qi* to stop vomiting; clearing manipulation on stomach-meridian point can strengthen the effect of descending adverse flow of *qi* to stop vomiting; arc-pushing *bagua* point clockwise is able to harmonize *qi*, dredge indigestion, harmonize *yin-yang*; clearing manipulation on heaven-river-water point is able to clear the heart and purge fire; pounding small-heaven-center point is able to relieve convulsion and tranquilize mind.

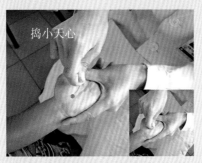

图 4 – 55　捣小天心
Picture 4 – 55　Pounding small-heaven-center point

101

预防与护理

1. 预防

（1）注意饮食卫生，不吃腐烂变质的食物，食用生、凉食品要新鲜。

（2）饮食有规律，按顿吃饭，不乱吃零食及饮料；不随心所欲，暴饮暴食；不嗜好生冷、辛辣无度，尽量避免饮食对胃黏膜的伤害。

（3）注意儿童的心理健康，尽量减少其心理压力，减轻学习负担，给儿童一个幸福、快乐的童年。

（4）酸、碱等有腐蚀性的化学物品应妥善保管，放到儿童不易取到的地方，以防误服。

（5）对胃有刺激性的药物尽量在饭后服用，减少对胃的刺激。

2. 家庭护理

（1）对于呕吐较重的患儿应禁食，病情缓解后再进流质、半流质、软食，减轻胃的负担，恢复脾胃功能；禁食肥甘、厚味、辛辣刺激及不易消化的食物。

（2）对于胃寒呕吐的患儿以散寒止痛为目的，轻症局部温熨，内服生姜红糖汤。饮食宜温，忌生冷瓜果。

（3）婴幼儿呕吐者必须加强护理，侧卧位，防止呕吐物吸到肺，引起窒息或吸入性肺炎。

（4）病愈后要饮食有节，给予高蛋白质、高维生素、营养丰富的食物。

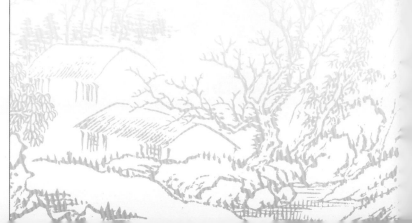

Prevention and Care

1 Prevention

1.1 Pay attention to food hygiene, do not eat spoiled food, and the raw, cool food should be fresh.

1.2 Eat regularly and do not eat snacks and drinks uncontrolledly. Do not eat too much nor cold and spicy food excessively. Try to avoid injury of food on the gastric mucosa.

1.3 Pay attention to children's mental health, try to minimize their psychological pressure, reduce the burden of their learning, and let children have a happy childhood.

1.4 The corrosive chemicals such as acid and alkali must be stored carefully out of reach of children in case the chemicals should be taken wrongly.

1.5 The irritant medicine for stomach should be taken after meals in order to reduce irritation for stomach.

2 Home care

2.1 For children with severe vomiting, fasting should be taken and the liquid, semi-liquid, and soft food can be eaten successively after remission to reduce the burden of the stomach and therefore restore the functions of the spleen and stomach. Fat, oversweet, greasy, spicy and indigestible foods are forbidden.

2.2 Relieving cold and pain is generally used for children with vomiting caused by stomach cold. Warm ironing therapy is applied topically in mild case, drinking brown sugar and ginger soup is recommended. Eat warm food, no raw or cold fruit.

2.3 Infants with vomiting must be cared carefully. Let the infant take lateral position to prevent choking or aspiration pneumonia caused by aspirating vomitus into the lungs.

2.4 After recovery, a moderate diet and high protein, high vitamin, nutrient-rich foods are recommended.

第五节　泄泻

　　泄泻是以大便次数增多，粪质稀薄或如水样为其主症。是小儿时期最常见的疾病之一，尤以 2 岁以下的婴幼儿更为常见，年龄愈小，发病率愈高。

病因病机

　　中医学认为，小儿脾胃薄弱，无论感受外邪，内伤乳食或脾肾虚弱等均可导致脾胃运化功能失调而发生泄泻。其主要的病变在于脾胃，因胃主腐熟水谷，脾主运化精微，如脾胃受病，则饮食入胃，水谷不化，精微不布，合污而下，致成泄泻。

　　小儿泄泻的原因，以感受外邪，内伤饮食和脾胃虚弱等为多见。小儿脏腑脆嫩，藩篱不密，易为外邪所侵，且因脾胃薄弱，不耐受邪，若脾受邪困，运化失职，升降失调，水谷不分，合污而下，则为泄泻；乳哺不当，饮食失节或过食生冷瓜果，或不消化食物，皆能损伤脾胃，脾伤则运化功能失职，胃伤则不能消磨水谷，宿食内停，清浊不分，并走大肠，因成泄泻；小儿先天禀赋不足，后天调护失宜，或久病迁延不愈，皆可导致脾胃虚弱。脾虚则健运失司，胃弱则不能腐熟水谷，因而水反为湿，谷反为滞，清阳不升，乃致合污而下，成为泄泻。

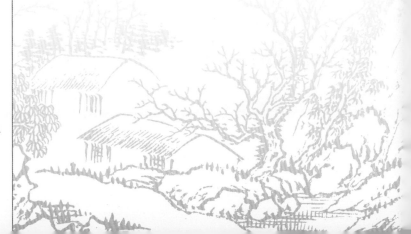

Section 5　Diarrhea

The main symptoms of diarrhea are increase of bowel movements with loose or watery stool. It is one of the most common diseases in infants, especially those below 2-year. The younger the age, the higher the incidence.

Cause and mechanism of disease

In TCM, infantile viscera are tender and weak in defending, so they are vulnerable to pathogens. It is so of spleen and stomach, whose normal transportation and transformation functions will be disturbed by external contraction, internal injury of infantile diet, or spleen and kidney deficiency, etc., leading to diarrhea.

The root of diarrhea is in stomach and spleen, because stomach governs digestion and spleen governs transportation and transformation of essence. If stomach and spleen are ill, the food we take will remain undigested, the essence will fail to be transported, and together with descending waste, there will be diarrhea.

Causes of infantile diarrhea are mainly in external contraction, internal injury of diet, and spleen and kidney deficiency.

If spleen is impaired by external contraction, it fails to have normal transportation and transformation functions, which results in disharmony of descending and ascending, dyspepsia, and together with descending waste, leading to diarrhea.

If stomach and spleen are impaired by internal injury of diet, such as improper breast feeding, irregular diet, overeating of raw and cold fruit, and indigestible food, the spleen will fail to have normal transportation and transformation functions while the stomach will fail to grind food. This will result in food stagnation, separation failure of the clear and turbid, and all the stuff go into large intestine, leading to diarrhea.

Infantile innate endowment is not enough, and together with improper nursing or chronic diseases, the spleen and stomach will be deficient. Deficient spleen fails to transport and deficient stomach fails to digest, and then, there will be dampness and food stagnation. As a result, it checks the ascending of clear *yang* and in blending with downward waste, leading to diarrhea.

105

辨证施治

1. 伤食泻

脘腹胀满，肚腹作痛，痛则欲泻，泻后痛减，粪便酸臭，或如败卵，嗳气酸馊，或欲呕吐，不思乳食，夜卧不安，舌苔厚腻。

辨证要点 脘腹胀满，痛则欲泻，泻后痛减，粪便酸臭，舌苔厚腻。

治则 清热导滞，和中止泻。

取穴 清胃 清天河水 运八卦 清补大肠（图4-56～图4-59）

方义 清胃经以消食化积，顺应升降；食积多有郁热，清天河水以清散郁热；顺运八卦可宽胸理气，消积导滞；清补大肠具有调理肠腑、渗湿止泻之功。

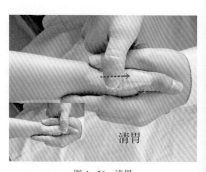

图4-56 清胃
Picture 4-56 Clearing manipulation on stomach-meridian point

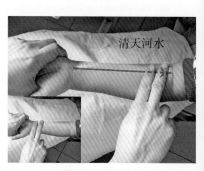

图4-57 清天河水
Picture 4-57 Clearing manipulation on heaven-river-water point

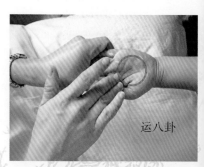

图4-58 运八卦
Picture 4-58 Arc-pushing *bagua* point

Treatment according to syndrome differentiation

1 Dyspeptic diarrhea

This diarrhea is characterized as distending and full stomach and abdomen, painful abdomen before bowel movements, pain relieved after bowel movements, acid and stinking stool or smelly stool as rotten eggs, acid belching or impulses of vomiting, no appetite for breast feeding, restless sleep, thick and greasy fur.

• Differentiation guidelines: distending and full stomach and abdomen, painful abdomen before bowel movements, pain relieved after bowel movements, acid and stinking stool, thick and greasy fur.

• Therapeutic principle: clearing heat and removing food stagnation, harmonizing middle *jiao* and stopping diarrhea.

• Treatment: clearing manipulation on stomach-meridian point and heaven-river-water point, arc-pushing *bagua* point, and pushing large-intestine-meridian point to and fro. (Picture 4−56 to Picture 4−59)

• Prescription analysis: Clearing manipulation on stomach-meridian point aims to promote digestion and remove food stagnation to follow the ascending and descending of the stomach *qi*; food stagnation often leads to stagnated heat, clearing heaven-river-water point is able to clear stagnated heat; arc-pushing *bagua* point clockwise can free chest and smooth *qi* flow, and remove food stagnation; pushing large-intestine-meridian point to and fro can regulate the large intestine, eliminate dampness and stop diarrhea.

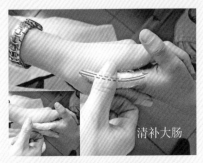

图 4−59 清补大肠
Picture 4−59 Pushing large-intestine-meridian
point to and fro

107

2．风寒泻

泄泻清稀，中多泡沫，臭气不甚，肠鸣腹痛，或兼恶寒发热，舌苔白腻。

辨证要点 泄泻清稀，中多泡沫，舌苔白腻。

治则 疏风散寒，温中止泻。

取穴 揉一窝风 揉外劳宫 清补大肠（图4-60～图4-62）

愈后以清补脾善后。

方义 揉一窝风以发散风寒；揉外劳宫温中散寒而止痛；清补大肠以调理肠腑，渗湿止泻。

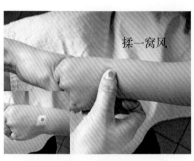

图4-60 揉一窝风
Picture 4-60 Kneading *yiwofeng* point

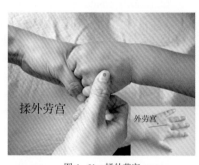

图4-61 揉外劳宫
Picture 4-61 Kneading dorsal-*laogong* point

3．湿热泻

泻下稀薄，水分较多，或如水注，粪色深黄而臭，或见少许黏液，腹部时感疼痛，食欲不振，肢体倦怠，发热或不发热，口渴，小便短黄，舌苔黄腻。

辨证要点 泻下稀薄，粪色深黄而臭，或见少许黏液，口渴，小便短黄，舌苔黄腻。

治则 清热利湿，和中止泻。

取穴 平肝 清胃 清天河水 清补大肠（图4-63～图4-65）

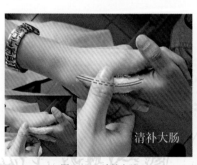

图4-62 清补大肠
Picture 4-62 Pushing large-intestine-meridian point to and fro

2 Wind-cold diarrhea

This diarrhea is characterized as thin and loose stool bearing with foam, not very smelly, borborygmus, pain in abdomen, or accompanied with fever and aversion to cold, whitish and greasy fur.

• Differentiation guidelines: thin and loose stool bearing with foam, whitish and greasy fur.

• Therapeutic principle: dredging wind and dispelling cold, warming middle *jiao* and stopping diarrhea.

• Treatment: kneading *yiwofeng* point and dorsal-*laogong* point, and pushing large-intestine-meridian point to and fro. (Picture 4 – 60 to Picture 4 – 62)

After the recovery from diarrhea, push spleen-meridian point to and fro for rehabilitation.

• Prescription analysis: Kneading *yiwofeng* point is able to diffuse wind and cold; kneading dorsal-*laogong* point can warm the middle *jiao* and dispel cold to stop pain; pushing large-intestine-meridian point to and fro aims to regulate the large intestine, eliminate dampness to stop diarrhea.

3 Damp-heat diarrhea

This diarrhea is characterized as thin stool with water in chief proportion or pouring watery stool, smelly and dark yellow stool with a bit of mucus, occasional pain in abdomen, no appetite, lassitude, fever or no fever, thirsty, short and yellow urine, yellowish and greasy fur.

• Differentiation guidelines: thin, smelly and dark yellow stool, or stool with a bit of mucus, thirsty, short and yellow urine, yellowish and greasy fur.

• Therapeutic principle: clearing heat and draining dampness, harmonizing middle *jiao* and stopping diarrhea.

• Treatment: clearing manipulation on liver-meridian point, stomach-meridian point, heaven-river-water point, and pushing large-intestine-meridian point to and fro. (Picture 4 – 63 to Picture 4 – 65)

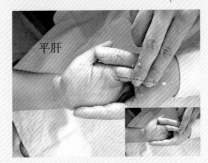

图 4 – 63 平肝

Picture 4 – 63 Clearing manipulation on liver-meridian point

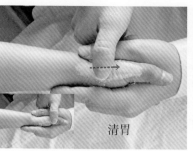

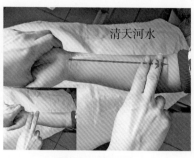

图 4-64　清胃
Picture 4-64　Clearing manipulation on
stomach-meridian point

图 4-65　清天河水
Picture 4-65　Clearing manipulation on heaven-
river-water point

方义　清肝经意在清泻肝火，行气导滞；清胃经意在清内湿热；清天河水可清一切热邪，以增强清热利湿之效；清补大肠以调理肠腑，渗湿止泻。

4. 脾虚泻

大便稀溏，多见食后作泻，色淡不臭，时轻时重，面色萎黄，肌肉消瘦，神疲倦怠，舌淡苔白。且易反复发作。

辨证要点　大便稀溏，多见食后作泻，面色萎黄，舌淡苔白，且易反复发作。

治则　健脾止泻。

取穴　清补大肠　清补脾　补脾（图 4-66～图 4-68）

方义　清补大肠经意在调理肠腑，化湿止泻；清补脾经意在健脾助运而止泻；补脾经意在健脾益气而止泻。

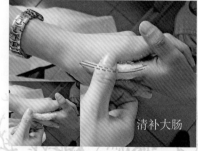

图 4-66　清补大肠
Picture 4-66　Pushing large-intestine-
meridian point to and fro

- Prescription analysis: Clearing manipulation on liver-meridian point is able to clear liver fire, promote *qi* flow and remove food stagnation; clearing manipulation on stomach-meridian point is able to expel damp and heat; clearing manipulation on heaven-river-water point can clear all kinds of heat evil, strengthen the effect of expelling damp and heat; pushing large-intestine-meridian point to and fro aims to regulate the large intestine, eliminate dampness to stop diarrhea.

4　Spleen-deficiency diarrhea

This diarrhea is characterized as loose stool, bowel movements soon after eating, pale color and not very smelly, sallow complexion, emaciating, listlessness, pale tongue, white fur and repeated occurrences.

- Differentiation guidelines: loose stool, bowel movements after eating, sallow complexion, pale tongue, white fur, and repeated occurrences.
- Therapeutic principle: invigorating spleen and stopping diarrhea.
- Treatment: pushing large-intestine-meridian and spleen-meridian point to and fro, nourishing manipulation on spleen-meridian point. (Picture 4 – 66 to Picture 4 – 68)
- Prescription analysis: Pushing large-intestine-meridian point to and fro aims to regulate the large intestine, eliminate dampness to stop diarrhea; pushing the spleen-meridian point to and fro is able to activate the spleen and aid in transportation to stop diarrhea; nourishing manipulation on spleen-meridian point aims to invigorate the spleen, replenish *qi* to stop diarrhea.

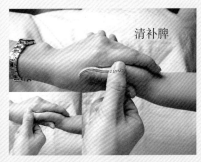 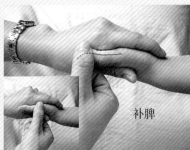

图 4 – 67　清补脾
Picture 4 – 67　Pushing spleen-meridian point to and fro

图 4 – 68　补脾
Picture 4 – 68　Nourishing manipulation on spleen-meridian point

预防与护理

1. 小儿泄泻重在预防，如何防止小儿腹泻的发生呢？

（1）**定量定时，调配合理**　人的饮食要有节制、有规律，它是保证小儿脾胃功能健全的基本措施。因此，小儿饮食必须定时定量，少吃零食，少量多餐，不要偏食、择食，防止进食过多或过少。

（2）**注意宜忌，保护脾胃**　由于小儿"脾常不足"，消化有限，但营养需求量大，为了不增加其胃肠负担，保证营养供给，小儿宜进清淡，细饮，易咀嚼，易消化，营养价值高的饮食，可选择适合小儿消化能力和符合营养的高蛋白质和各种新鲜蔬菜及水果，凡辛辣刺激、生冷瓜果、油腻、坚硬难化之物均须慎忌。

（3）**讲究卫生，防病入口**　小儿胃肠抵抗力差，病邪容易从口而入，所以必须注意食物新鲜、清洁，同时养成小儿良好的饮食卫生习惯，饭前便后洗手，细嚼慢咽，不宜用手抓饭或口对口喂食，此外，防止进食时嬉闹。

2. 小儿腹泻时应如何护理？

（1）对感染性腹泻儿应注意消毒隔离，对其排泄物进行消毒处理；注意小儿呕吐、排便和排尿的量，以便及时补足丢失的水分；睡眠时采取侧卧位，以免呕吐物误吸引起窒息或肺炎；加强臀部护理，勤换尿布，大便后冲洗臀部，以防引起尿布疹、臀部感染和尿路感染。

（2）**喂养方面**

A. 腹泻时由于肠道的吸收功能减弱和由于呕吐使进食量减少易导致小儿营养不良，所以在腹泻时足够的营养供给对保证疾病恢复、减少体重下降和生长发育停滞的程度十分重要。重度脱水伴呕吐者可暂禁食4～6小时，应继续给予饮食。因为担心进食会引起大便次数、量增多而给予禁食是不适宜的。

Prevention and Care

1 Prevention is very important. How to prevent diarrhea in children?

1.1 Quantitative and timing, a reasonable diet: A moderate, regular diet is essential measures for babies to ensure their healthy function of the stomach. So the baby's diet should be quantitative and timing, little snacks, frequent meals with less quantity, no food preferences, and not eating too much or too little.

1.2 Paying attention to food prohibition and protecting the spleen and stomach: Babies should be fed a light, fine, easy to chew and digest diet with high nutritional value in order not to increase the burden of the stomach and to ensure the supply of nutrients on the ground that the function of the spleen in babies is often inadequate and its digestion is limited while their demand for nutrition is big. Select suitable diet according to the baby's ability to digest, such as high nutritional value diet, a variety of fresh vegetables and fruits. Spicy, raw, greasy, hard and indigestible food or fruits are not recommended.

1.3 Paying attention to hygiene and preventing illness from entering by the mouth: Pediatric gastrointestinal duct has poor resistance, pathogenic factors easily go into the body from the mouth, Let children take fresh and clean food and develop good habits of food hygiene, such as washing hands before eating and after relieving, eating slowly, not eating rice with hand or mouth-feeding, and preventing eating when frolicking.

2 How to care for the baby with diarrhea?

2.1 For the baby with infectious diarrhea, such measures as disinfection and isolation should be taken like the disinfection about excreta. Pay attention the baby's volume of vomiting, defecation and urination to make up for the loss of water promptly and let the baby take a lateral position during sleep in order to avoid suffocation or pneumonia caused by aspirating vomitus. Pay more attention to the hip care including frequently changing the diapers, washing buttocks after relieving to prevent diaper rash, hip infections and urinary tract infections.

2.2 Feeding

2.2.1 Weak absorptive function of the intestines due to diarrhea and reduced food intaking due to vomiting easily cause infantile malnutrition

113

B.母乳喂养者应持续给予母乳喂养；人工喂养者在 6 个月以内可给予病儿日常食用的奶制品略加水稀释或给予等量的米汤，随腹泻好转逐渐恢复到正常饮食，6 个月以上者给予平常已经习惯了的饮食，如米粥、面条、蔬菜、鱼或肉末等。可给予一些新鲜水果汁或水果以补充维生素和钾。

C.腹泻停止后，继续给予营养丰富的饮食，并可每日加餐 1 次，直到腹泻停止后 2 周，以期赶上正常生长。营养不良儿或慢性腹泻儿的恢复期更长，加餐可直到营养不良恢复。

第六节 腹痛

腹痛是一个证候，引起腹痛的原因很多，如外感、饮食、情绪以及脏腑功能失调的种种因素，都是诱发腹痛的重要原因，而其临床表现复杂，涉及面广，因此临症时必须详细了解病情，并全面考虑。在此，首先除外器质性疾病。

中医学认为，腹痛是指胃脘以下，耻骨毛际以上的部位发生疼痛的一种病证，其多因外感、内伤影响了脏腑经脉的正常功能，导致脏腑经脉气机郁滞不通，气血运行受阻或气血不足失于温养，发生腹痛。

病因病机

小儿腹痛的主要原因可概括为以下几方面。

1. 乳食积滞

因乳食不节，过食油腻厚味，或暴饮强食，临卧多食，以致食积停滞，郁积胃肠，气机壅塞，痞满膜胀而腹痛。小儿饮食不能自节，脾胃运化功能薄弱，因而乳食停滞，损伤脾胃，是小儿腹痛的主要原因之一。

and therefore it is very important to provide the sick with adequate supply of nutrients to ensure his/her recovery from illness, reduce the severity of weight loss and growth stagnation. With regard to the baby with severe dehydration with vomiting, temporary fasting for 4-6 hours may be given and then taking food is preferred. Fasting is not appropriate because of the worry about increased frequency and amount of defecation caused by eathing.

2.2.2   For the breastfed baby, continuing breastfeeding is preferred; for the artificial fed baby six months or below, the daily dairy products diluted with water slightly or the same amount of rice soup is appropriate. With his/her recovery, the baby can be fed a normal diet. For the baby over 6 months is given a normal diet as usual, such as rice, noodles, vegetables, fish or minced meat and so on. Some fresh fruit juices or fruits can be fed to supplement vitamins and potassium.

2.2.3   After the diarrhea stops, continue to provide nutritious diet and an extra meal daily for two weeks to make the baby grow normally. The baby with malnutrition or chronic diarrhea needs more time to recover, an extra meal discontinues until his /her malnutrition disappears.

Section 6   Abdominal Pain

Abdominal pain is a syndrome of pain in abdomen caused by external contraction, diet, emotions, and disharmony of viscera. Its clinical manifestation is not only complicated, but also has a wide range of involvement, which requires detailed understanding of the state of the disease and an overall consideration. Physical illnesses should be excluded at first.

In TCM, abdominal pain refers to the syndrome of pain in the region below stomach area and above the hairy area of pubis. In most cases, abdominal pain is caused by external contraction and internal injury, which affects the normal function of viscera and meridians, leading to stagnated *qi* movements of viscera and meridians, obstructed circulation of *qi* and blood, or insufficient *qi* and blood to warm and nourish.

Cause and mechanism of disease

There are five chief causes of infant abdominal pain.

1   Stagnation of milk and food

Irregular eating of milk and food, over eating of oily, greasy and heavy

115

2. 感受寒邪

由于人们生活水平的提高，冰箱极为普及，加之对独生子女的溺爱，过食生冷者居多，另外，护理不当，风冷寒邪侵入脐腹，肠胃受冷，中阳受伐，寒凝则气滞，气滞则经脉不通，以致气机不畅，气血壅阻而腹痛。由于小儿稚阳之体，腹痛因于寒者居多。

3. 燥热内结

平素过食辛辣香燥，膏粱厚味，胃肠积热，或积滞日久化热，肠中津液不足，形成燥热闭结，或因外感病，热邪传里，热结阳明，灼伤津液，使气机失于疏利，传导之令不行而致腹痛。

4. 气滞血瘀

由于生活节奏的增快，家长望子成龙心切，学龄儿童心理压力增加，久之则肝气不疏，郁而化火，肝郁气滞则脾土受伐；或因脏腑娇嫩，成而未全，全而未壮，神气怯弱，对外界突如其来的刺激，缺乏综合分析能力，容易引起气血逆乱，脏腑气机不畅，气血运行受阻而引起腹痛。

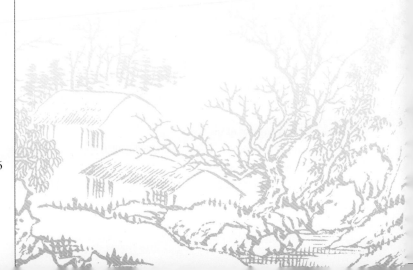

flavored food, too much drinking and eating, or too much eating before sleep can cause stagnation of milk and food in stomach and intestine. Then *qi* movement is clogged up, engendering abdominal distension, and leading to abdominal pain. Because infant is incapable of self-regulating diet, and the spleen and stomach are vulnerable, so this is one of the chief causes of infant abdominal pain

2 Invasion of cold-evil

As the refrigerator is a necessity in daily life, parents tend to neglect the raw and cold food are bad for infants. In addition with improper nursing, wind-cold invades navel, through which the stomach and intestine catch cold, and the *yang qi* in the middle *jiao* is impaired. When cold congeals, *qi* stagnates. When *qi* stagnates, meridians are obstructed. The result is *qi* movement fails to run smoothly, circulation of *qi* and blood is blocked, leading to abdominal pain. Infant *yang* is immature, so most cases of abdominal pain are due to the catch of cold-evil.

3 Constipation of dryness-heat

Over eating of heavy flavored food, such as acrid, scented, dry and greasy food, may result in heat accumulation in stomach and intestine. A long time of food stagnation will also engendering heat, which boils the fluid of intestine to insufficient, leading to constipation of dryness-heat. Moreover, when external contraction invades, heat evil goes into the body and accumulates in *yangming* meridians, which burns fluid, and makes *qi* movement fail to dredge. Constipation of dryness-heat contributes to the failure of large intestine to convey, leading to abdominal pain.

4 *Qi* stagnation and blood stasis

As expectations from parents are high, the psychological pressure of children of schooling age is increasing, and if it haunts for a long time, their liver *qi* will be constrained and stagnated, ultimately impairing spleen. Moreover, infantile viscera are tender and immature, so when there are abrupt external stimulants, they are easily affected and have adverse rising *qi* and blood, disturbance of visceral *qi* movement, or blocked *qi* and blood, leading to abdominal pain.

117

5. 脏腑虚寒

常见于素体阳虚或病后体弱，脾胃虚寒，脾阳不能温运，以致寒湿内停，气机不畅，气血不足，失于温养，而致腹部隐隐作痛。

辨证施治

1. 食积腹痛

脘腹胀满，疼痛拒按，不思乳食，嗳腐吞酸或腹痛欲泻，泻后痛减，时有呕吐，吐物酸馊，夜卧不安，时时啼哭，苔多厚腻。

辨证要点　脘腹胀满，疼痛拒按，不思乳食，夜卧不安，时时啼哭，苔多厚腻。

治则　消食，清热，止痛。

取穴　平肝　清胃　清大肠　运八卦（图4-69~图4-72）

方义　平肝经意在疏肝理气而止痛；清胃经以和胃消食化积；清大肠经有通导积滞之功；顺运八卦有宽胸理气之功，气机通畅，疼痛自止。

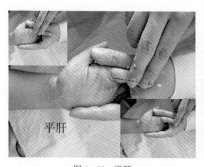

图4-69　平肝
Picture 4-69　Clearing manipulation on liver-meridian point

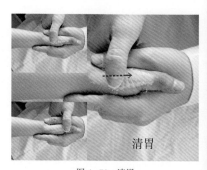

图4-70　清胃
Picture 4-70　Clearing manipulation on stomach-meridian point

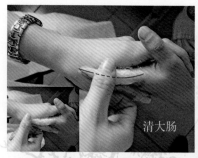

图4-71　清大肠
Picture 4-71　Clearing manipulation on large-intestine-meridian point

5   Cold-deficiency viscera

It is common among infants who have *yang* deficiency physique or those who are weak after a long period of illness. When spleen and stomach are in a cold-deficiency state, spleen *yang* fails to have the function of warming and transportation. Resultantly, there will be cold-damp retention, disturbance of *qi* movement, deficient *qi* and blood, and lack of warming, leading to looming pain in abdomen.

Treatment according to syndrome differentiation

1   Abdominal pain of food stagnation

This abdominal pain is characterized as fullness and stuffiness in stomach and abdomen, pain aggravated by pressing, no appetite, belching and acid regurgitation, or diarrhea synchronized with abdominal pain, pain relieved after diarrhea, vomiting with acid and smelly contents, restless sleep, frequent to cry, thick and greasy fur.

- Differentiation guidelines: fullness and stuffiness in stomach and abdomen, pain aggravated by pressing, no appetite, restless sleep, frequent cry, thick and greasy fur.

- Therapeutic principle: promoting digestion, clearing heat, and stopping pain.

- Treatment: clearing manipulation on liver-meridian point, stomach-meridian point and large-intestine-meridian point, and arc-pushing *bagua* point. (Picture 4-69 to Picture 4-72)

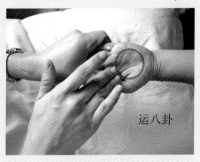

图 4-72　运八卦
Picture 4-72　Arc-pushing *bagua* point

- Prescription analysis: clearing manipulation on liver-meridian point aims to relieve the pain by soothing the liver and regulating the *qi*; clearing manipulation on stomach-meridian point can promote digestion and remove food stagnation by harmonizing stomach; clearing the large-intestine-meridian point can dredge and discharge indigestion; arc-pushing *bagua* point clockwise can free chest and smooth *qi* flow and pain will disappear after *qi* flow is smooth.

2．寒积腹痛

腹部疼痛，阵阵发作，痛处喜暖，得温则舒，遇寒痛甚，肠鸣辘辘，或兼吐泻。痛甚者，额冷汗出，面色苍白，唇色紫暗，手足发凉，舌淡红，苔多白滑。

辨证要点 腹痛较甚，痛处喜暖，得温则舒，舌淡苔白。

治则 温中散寒，理气止痛。

取穴 揉一窝风 揉外劳宫 揉板门 运八卦（图4-73～图4-76）

方义 揉一窝风散寒理气而止痛；揉外劳宫温中助阳而散寒；揉板门具有通调三焦气机之功；顺运八卦调理脏腑之气血，气血通畅则痛止。

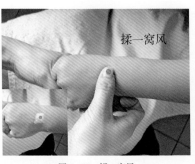

揉一窝风

图4-73 揉一窝风
Picture 4-73　Kneading *yiwofeng* point

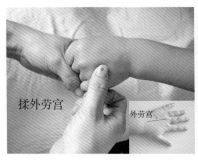

揉外劳宫

外劳宫

图4-74 揉外劳宫
Picture 4-74　Kneading dorsal-*laogong* point

3．实热腹痛

腹痛胀满，疼痛拒按，潮热，大便秘结，烦躁口渴，手足心热，唇红舌红，苔黄燥。

辨证要点 腹痛拒按，大便秘结，手足心热，舌红苔黄燥。

治则 通腑泄热，行气止痛。

取穴 平肝 清胃 退六腑 揉板门（图4-77～图4-80）

方义 平肝经意在疏肝理气而止痛；清胃经清泻胃肠积热，与退六腑共奏通腑泄热而止痛之功；揉板门具有通调三焦气机之功，气机通畅则痛止。

2　Abdominal pain of cold accumulation

This abdominal pain is characterized as intermittent pain in abdomen, pain relieved by warm and aggravated by cold, accelerated borborygmus, or with vomiting and diarrhea together, cold and sweating forehead in serious pain, pale complexion, dark purple lips, cold limbs, pale-red tongue, white and slippery fur.

- Differentiation guidelines: intermittent and severe pain in abdomen, warming favors in the pain region, pain relieved by warmth, pale-red tongue, and white fur.
- Therapeutic principle: warming middle *jiao* and dispelling cold, regulating *qi* movement and stopping pain.
- Treatment: kneading *yiwofeng* point, dorsal-*laogong* point, and *banmen* point, arc-pushing *bagua* point. (Picture 4－73 to Picture 4－76)
- Prescription analysis: Kneading *yiwofeng* point aims to expel cold, smooth *qi* flow to stop pain; kneading dorsal-*laogong* point can warm the middle *jiao* and aid in *yang* to dispel cold; kneading *banmen* point can harmonize *qi* activity of the *sanjiao*; arc-pushing *bagua* point clockwise aims to stop pain by harmonizing *qi* and blood of *zang-fu organs*.

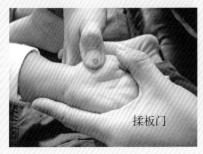
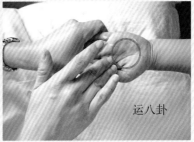

图 4－75　揉板门
Picture 4－75　Kneading *banmen* point

图 4－76　运八卦
Picture 4－76　Arc-pushing *bagua* point

3　Abdominal pain of excess heat

The abdominal pain is characterized as pain and fullness in abdomen, pain aggravated by pressing, tidal fever, constipation, restlessness, thirsty, heat sensation in palms and soles, red lips and tongue, yellow and dry fur.

- Differentiation guidelines: abdominal pain aggravated by pressing, constipation, heat sensation in palms and soles, red tongue, yellow and dry fur.

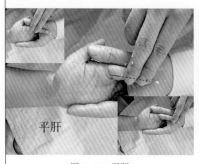

平肝

图 4-77 平肝
Picture 4-77 Clearing manipulation on liver-meridian point

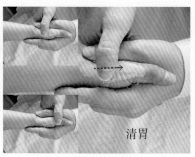

清胃

图 4-78 清胃
Picture 4-78 Clearing manipulation on stomach-meridian point

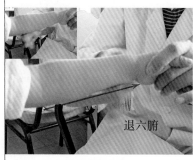

退六腑

图 4-79 退六腑
Picture 4-79 Clearing manipulation on six-*fu* point

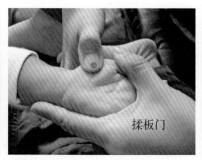

揉板门

图 4-80 揉板门
Picture 4-80 Kneading *banmen* point

4．气滞腹痛

脘腹胀痛，走窜攻冲，痛引两胁，或痛引小腹，疼痛多于晨起发作，嗳气或矢气则痛减，舌淡苔薄。

辨证要点 腹痛游走不定，多于晨起发生，嗳气或矢气则痛减。

治则 理气止痛。

取穴 平肝 运八卦 推四横纹 揉板门（图 4-81～图 4-84）

方义 平肝经疏肝理气而止痛；顺运八卦调理脏腑之气血；推四横纹能消食化积，理气止痛；揉板门具有通调三焦气机之功，脏腑气血通畅则腹痛自止。

• Therapeutic principle: opening *fu* organs to purging heat, promoting *qi* flow to relieve pain.

• Treatment: clearing manipulation on liver-meridian point, stomach-meridian point and six-*fu* point, and kneading *banmen* point. (Picture 4 – 77 to Picture 4 – 80)

• Prescription analysis: Clearing manipulation on liver-meridian point aims to relieve the pain by soothing the liver and regulating the *qi*; clearing manipulation on stomach-meridian point and six-*fu* point to stop pain by resolving stagnated heat in the stomach and intestines; kneading *banmen* point can stop pain by smoothing *qi* activity in the *sanjiao*.

4   Abdominal pain of *qi* stagnation

This abdominal pain is characterized as distending and wandering pain and fullness in stomach and abdomen, sometimes radiating pain to hypochondriac region or lower abdomen, usually morning pain, pain relieved by belching or flatus, pale tongue and thin fur.

• Differentiation guidelines: wandering abdominal pain, usually morning pain, pain relieved by belching or flatus.

• Therapeutic principle: regulating *qi* movement to relieve pain.

• Treatment: clearing manipulation on liver-meridian point, arc-pushing *bagua* point, pushing four-transverse-crease point, and kneading *banmen* point. (Picture 4 – 81 to Picture 4 – 84)

• Prescription analysis: Clearing manipulation on liver-meridian point aims to relieve the pain by soothing the liver and regulating the *qi*; arc-

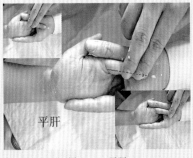

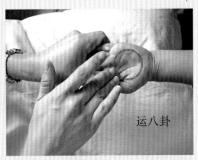

图 4 – 81   平肝
Picture 4 – 81   Clearing manipulation on liver-meridian point

图 4 – 82   运八卦
Picture 4 – 82   Arc-pushing *bagua* point

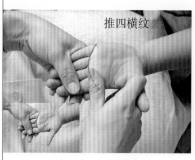

推四横纹

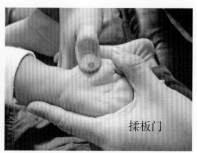

揉板门

图4-83 推四横纹
Picture 4-83 Pushing four-transverse-crease
point

图4-84 揉板门
Picture 4-84 Kneading *banmen* point

5．虚寒腹痛

腹痛绵绵，时作时止，痛处喜温喜按，面色苍白，精神倦怠，手足清冷，饮食较少，或食后作胀，大便稀溏，唇舌淡白。

辨证要点　腹痛时作时止，痛处喜温喜按，伴有脾虚症状。

治则　温中健脾止痛。

取穴　揉外劳宫　清补脾　揉板门　推四横纹（图4-85～图4-88）

方义　揉外劳宫以温阳散寒而止痛；清补脾经以健脾助运而达到消积止痛的目的；揉板门能通达气机，顺其升降而止痛；推四横纹能化积行气而止痛。

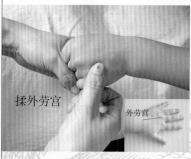

揉外劳宫

外劳宫

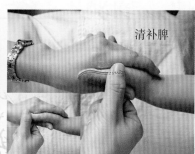

清补脾

图4-85 揉外劳宫
Picture 4-85 Kneading dorsal-*laogong* point

图4-86 清补脾
Picture 4-86 Pushing spleen-meridian point to
and fro

pushing *bagua* point clockwise aims to stop pain by harmonizing *qi* and blood of *zang-fu* organ; pushing four-transverse-crease point can promote digestion, resolve food stagnation and relieve the pain by smoothing *qi* flow; kneading *banmen* point can stop pain by smoothing *qi* activity in the *sanjiao*.

5　Abdominal pain of cold-deficiency

This abdominal pain is characterized as looming abdominal pain, pain relieved by warming and pressing, pale complexion, lassitude, cold limbs, no appetite, or abdominal distension after eating, loose stool, pale tongue and lips.

- Differentiation guidelines: intermittent abdominal pain, pain relieved by warming and pressing, accompanied with syndrome of spleen deficiency.
- Therapeutic principle: warming middle *jiao*, invigorating spleen and relieving pain.
- Treatment: kneading dorsal-*laogong* point, pushing spleen-meridian point to and fro, kneading *banmen* point, and pushing four-transverse-crease point. (Picture 4 – 85 to Picture 4 – 88)
- Prescription analysis: Kneading dorsal-*laogong* point can stop pain by warming *yang* and expelling cold; pushing spleen-meridian point to and fro aims to remove food stagnation and stop pain by invigorating the spleen and aiding in transportation; kneading *banmen* point can stop pain by dredging and smoothing *qi* flow to follow the ascending and descending of *qi*; pushing four-transverse-crease point is able to stop pain by resolving food stagnation and smooth *qi* flow.

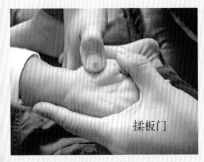
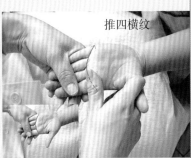

推四横纹

揉板门

图 4 – 87　揉板门
Picture 4 – 87　Kneading *banmen* point

图 4 – 88　推四横纹
Picture 4 – 88　Pushing four-transverse-crease point

125

预防与护理

（1）不合理的饮食习惯是导致腹痛的主要原因，因此，小儿在饮食方面应注意，不过食生冷瓜果，不过食油腻、煎炸之品，多食新鲜蔬菜。

（2）大量研究表明，疼痛不仅是一种感觉，它还涉及心理与行为的成分。因此，家长不要过分关注腹痛现象，因为反复发作性的腹痛有时与家长不适当的语言强化行为有关。

（3）避免感受寒邪，注意腹部保暖；饭后稍事休息，勿做剧烈运动，以利于胃肠消化、吸收。

（4）剧烈腹痛或腹痛不止者，随时检查腹部体征，尽早明确诊断，及时处理。

第七节　便秘

便秘是指排便时间延长（超过 48 小时）或粪质干燥难解的一种病证，可单独存在，也可继发于其他疾病过程中。

病因病机

中医学认为，饮食入胃，经脾的运化，吸收其精华，所剩糟粕，在肝的疏泄功能作用下，由大肠传送而出，肾开窍于二阴而主水液，司二便，故便秘虽病在大肠传导功能失职，却与脾胃、肝、肾诸脏也有密切关系，小儿胃肠脆弱，若乳食积滞，传导受阻；或燥热内结，肠液干涸；或肝脾郁结，气滞不行；或血亏、阴虚，肠失濡润；或气虚、阳虚，肠失温煦，传送无力，均可使大肠传导失职而致便秘。

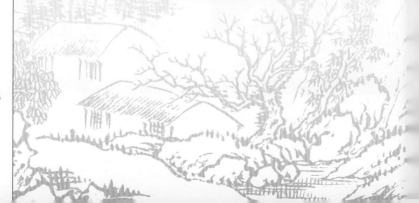

Prevention and Care

1 Unreasonable eating habit is the main cause of abdominal pain. So attention should be paid to the diet of baby. Do not eat either raw melon & fruit or greasy, fried food too much, eat fresh vegetables more.

2 Many studies show that pain is not only a feeling, but also affected by psychology and behavior. Therefore, parents should not be too concerned about the pain. Sometimes, some recurrent abdominal pain is related to the parent's inappropriate language.

3 Avoid catching cold pathogen, keep abdomen warm; take a break after a meal, do not do strenuous exercise in order to facilitate the digestion and absorption of the gastrointestine.

4 For severe or continued abdominal pain, check the abdominal physical signs at any time, make diagnosis as early as possible and treat it promptly.

Section 7　Constipation

Constipation is a kind of disease with prolonged interval of every two bowel movements (>48h) or difficult and dry stool. It may exist singly, or may be a symptom in the course of other diseases.

Cause and mechanism of disease

In TCM, the food taken is stored in stomach and through transportation and transformation functions of the spleen, the essence is absorbed and the waste, with the help of the dredging function of liver, is conveyed by the large intestine. Moreover, kidney controls urine and stool, because it opens into vulva and anus, and governs fluid. Thus, although constipation is ultimately attributed to the failure of large intestine to convey, it is closely related to the spleen, stomach, liver and kidney.

Infantile intestine and stomach are immature. If there is food and milk stagnation, the tract of conveys will be blocked. If there is dryness-heat retention, intestine fluid will be burned to deficient. If there is stagnation of spleen and liver *qi*, *qi* movement will be clogged. If there is blood deficiency or *yin* deficiency, intestine will be malnourished. If there is *qi* deficiency, *yang* deficiency, then the intestine will not warm itself and fail to convey. All these result in the failure of large intestine to convey, leading to constipation.

127

辨证施治

1. 虚寒便秘

神疲乏力，面色㿠白，时有便意，大便不干硬，但努挣乏力，用力则汗出短气，便后疲乏，舌淡苔薄。

辨证要点　排便时间延长，排便困难，但粪质不干硬，便后疲乏，舌淡苔薄。

治则　温阳益气，润肠通便。

取穴　揉外劳宫　清补脾　清补大肠（图4-89～图4-91）

方义　揉外劳宫温阳散寒；清补脾经具有健脾益气助运之功；清补大肠经可调理气机，以恢复正常的排便功能。

2. 实热便秘

大便干结，排出困难，或腹胀不适，兼呕吐，或口臭唇疮，面赤身热，苔黄燥。

辨证要点　大便干结，排出困难，面赤身热，苔黄燥。

治则　清热润肠通便。

取穴　平肝　清胃　退六腑　清大肠（图4-92～图4-95）

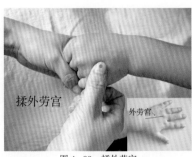

图4-89　揉外劳宫
Picture 4-89　Kneading dorsal-*laogong* point

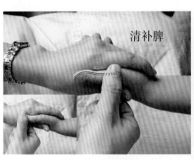

图4-90　清补脾
Picture 4-90　Pushing spleen-meridian point to and fro

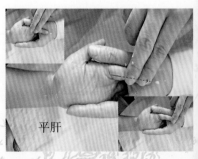

图4-92　平肝
Picture 4-92　Clearing manipulation on liver-meridian point

Treatment according to syndrome differentiation

1　Cold-deficiency constipation

It is characterized as lassitude, pale complexion, frequent awareness of defecation, loose stool, but lack of strength to pass stool, sweating and short of breath after exerting effort, tiresome after bowel movement, pale tongue and thin fur.

● Differentiation guidelines: prolonged duration of bowel movements, difficult and loose stool, tiresome after bowel movement, pale tongue and thin fur.

● Therapeutic principle: warming *Yang* and replenishing *qi*, moistening intestines and inducing stool.

● Treatment: kneading dorsal-*laogong* point, pushing spleen-meridian point to and fro, and pushing large-intestine-meridian point to and fro. (Picture 4 – 89 to Picture 4 – 91)

● Prescription analysis: Kneading dorsal-*laogong* point aims to warm *yang* and expel cold; pushing spleen-meridian point to and fro can activate the spleen, replenish *qi* and aid in transportation; pushing large-intestine-meridian point to and fro can harmonize *qi* activity in order to restore normal bowel movement.

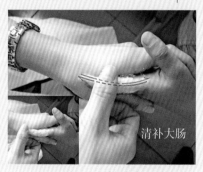

图 4-91　清补大肠
Picture 4 – 91　Pushing large-intestine-meridian point to and fro

2　Heat-excess constipation

It is characterized as dry and difficult stool, abdominal distension, accompanied with vomiting, smelly mouth, labial sores, flushed face, feverish sensation, dry and yellow fur.

● Differentiation guidelines: dry and difficult stool, flushed face, feverish sensation, dry and yellow fur.

● Therapeutic principle: clearing heat, moistening intestines and inducing stool.

● Treatment: clearing manipulation on liver-meridian point, stomach-meridian point, six-*fu* point, and large-intestine-meridian point. (Picture 4 – 92 to Picture 4 – 95)

129

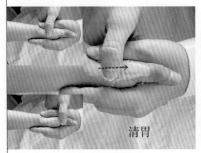
清胃

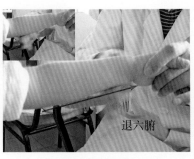
退六腑

图 4－93　清胃
Picture 4－93　Clearing manipulation on stomach-meridian point

图 4－94　退六腑
Picture 4－94　Clearing manipulation on six-*fu* point

　　方义　平肝经具有疏肝理气、顺气行滞以达排便之功能；清胃经可清泻胃火以消口臭而降气；退六腑具有清脏腑郁热、导滞通便的作用；清大肠经可荡涤肠腑邪热，达到热泄便通的目的。

预防与护理

　　（1）首先从饮食入手　应喂饱婴儿，较大婴儿合理给予蛋白质饮食，增加谷类食物，儿童多吃蔬菜、水果，多饮水，最好每日早晨起床后喝一杯蜂蜜水，使粪便柔软润滑，易于排出。

　　（2）训练定时排便　孩子应从小被训练在固定时间排便，定时坐便盆，养成按时排便的习惯，使直肠的排便运动产生条件反射。

　　（3）避免经常使用泻药　因为泻药虽有暂时通便作用，但久用之后，反而更减缓肠道蠕动，加重便秘。但对于疾病引起的肠壁肌肉张力减低、蠕动减慢者，应积极治疗原发病。

　　（4）病后护理　热病之后，由于进食甚少而多日未大便，不必急以通便，只需扶养胃气，待饮食渐增，大便自能正常。

• Prescription analysis: Clearing manipulation on liver-meridian point can smooth the liver and regulate *qi* flow, resolve food stagnation and promote bowel function; clearing manipulation on stomach-meridian point can clear stomach fire and eliminate bad breath to descend the adverse flow of *qi*; clearing manipulation on six-*fu* point is able to clear stagnated heat in the *zang-*

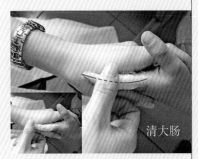

清大肠

图 4-95　清大肠
Picture 4-95　Clearing manipulation on large-intestine-meridian point

fu organs and remove stagnation by purgation; clearing manipulation on large-intestine-meridian point can relax bowels and discharge heat in the intestine.

Prevention and Care

1 Starting with feeding: Infants should be fed, the older baby can have protein diet and cereal, children can have more vegetables and fruits, and drink more water, they'd better drink a cup of honey water daily in the morning after getting up, and then the stool will be soft and smooth, easy to discharge.

2 Regular bowel movement training: Children should be trained to defecate in a fixed time from childhood, regularly use potty, develop the habit of regular bowel movement, and make bowel movement of the rectum develop a conditioned reflex.

3 Avoid frequent use of laxatives: Laxatives have laxative effect temporarily, but prolonged use of it will slow the peristalsis of the intestinal canal and worsen constipation. For reduced intestinal muscle tension and slow peristalsis caused by diseases, the primary disease should be treated actively.

4 Aftercare: After the fever, it is unnecessary to defecate hastily because of eating too little and having no bowel movement for several days. Just nourish stomach *qi*, appetite will gradually become better, and therefore bowel movement will be normal.

第八节　厌食症

厌食症是指小儿较长时期见食不贪，食欲不振，甚则拒食的一种常见病证。发病原因主要在于饮食喂养不当，导致脾胃不和，受纳运化失健。本症多见于1～6岁小儿。若因外感或某些慢性疾病而出现的食欲不振者，则不属本病范围。

病因病机

中医学认为，本症的主要原因，在于平素饮食不节，或因喂养不当，以及长期偏食等情况，损伤脾胃正常的运化功能，从而产生见食不贪，肌肉消瘦，影响正常的生长发育。小儿时期"脾常不足"，饮食不能自调，食物不知饥饱。有些家长缺乏育婴保健知识，片面强调给以高营养的滋补食物，超越了脾胃正常的运化能力，以及过于溺爱，或恣意投其所好，养成偏食习惯，或进食不定时，生活不规律等，皆可导致脾失健运，胃不思纳，脾胃不和的厌食症。

脾与胃互为表里，虽各有所司，但相互关联。如脾主运化，输布营养精微，升清降浊，为气血生化之源，五脏六腑、四肢百骸，皆赖之以养；胃主受纳、腐熟水谷，传于小肠，分清泌浊。两者在功能上虽各有所主，而彼此均互为影响。脾为阴土，喜燥而恶湿，得阳则运；胃为阳土，喜润而恶燥，以阴为用。故饮食失调，必伤脾胃，胃阴伤则不思进食，脾阳伤则运化失职。

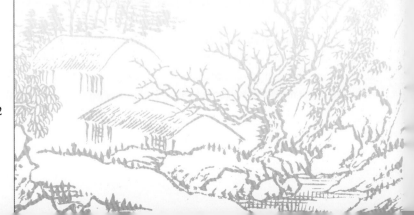

Section 8　Anorexia

Anorexia is a kind of disease in which children have no appetite, or even aversion to food for a long time. It is a common disease among infants in the year between 1 to 6. The chief cause is an improper feeding, which results in disharmony of spleen and stomach, and malfunctions of intake and transportation. Anorexia caused by external contraction or some chronic diseases is not discussed here.

Cause and mechanism of disease

In TCM, the causes of anorexia are an irregular diet, an improper feeding and dietary bias for a long time, by which the normal functions of transformation and transportation will be affected. Resultantly, there will be symptoms as loss of appetite, emaciation and influenced growth and development.

Infant has immature spleen and is unable to self-control diet, not knowing satiation and hunger. However, some parents lack the knowledge of nursing infants. They offer food of high nourishment, which more than often are unbearable for the normal functions of infantile spleen and stomach. In addition, infants are spoiled. They always get whatever they want and gradually become picky in eating. Also, irregular diet and life style may result in the failure of spleen in transportation and stomach in intake, leading to anorexia of spleen and stomach in disharmony.

Spleen governs transportation and transformation, and by spreading essence, sending up the fresh *qi* and lowering down the dross, it is the generation and transformation source of *qi* and blood. All parts of the body are dependent on the nourishment of spleen. Stomach governs intake and digestion, through which the digested food is conveyed to small intestine for separating the clear and turbid. Even though spleen and stomach have individual functions, they influence each other, in exterior and interior relation. Spleen pertains to *yin*-earth, which is in favor of dryness and in aversion to dampness, and it functions by the help of *yang*. Stomach pertains to *yang*-earth, which is in favor of moisture and in aversion to dryness, and it functions by the help of *yin*. So, if the diet is irregular, spleen and stomach will be impaired. Impairment of stomach *yin* results in no appetite while impairment of spleen *yang* results in the failure of transformation and transportation.

133

辨证施治

1. 脾运失健

面色少华，不思纳食，或食物无味，拒进饮食，形体偏瘦，而精神状态一般无特殊异常，大小便均基本正常，舌苔白或薄腻。

辨证要点　精神、活动正常，不思纳食，形态偏瘦，舌淡苔薄白。

治则　调胃和中，健脾助运。

取穴　清胃　清补脾　推四横纹（图4-96～图4-98）

方义　清胃经可开胃消食而化积；清补脾经可健脾益气而助运化；推四横纹以行气消积而增进食欲。

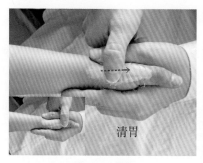

图4-96　清胃
Picture 4-96　Clearing manipulation on stomach-meridian point

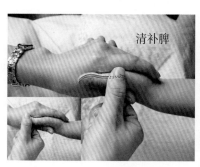

图4-97　清补脾
Picture 4-97　Pushing spleen-meridian point to and fro

2. 胃阴不足

口干多饮而不喜进食，皮肤干燥，缺乏润泽，大便多干结。舌苔多见光剥，质偏红。

辨证要点　口干欲饮不欲食，舌质偏红，多见光剥。

治则　养胃育阴。

取穴　清胃　清补脾　揉二马（图4-99～图4-101）

方义　清胃经可开胃消食而化积；清补脾经可健脾益气而助运化；揉二马滋阴养胃而助消化。

Treatment according to syndrome differentiation

1　Failure of splenic transportation

It is characterized as lusterless complexion, no appetite, or tasteless, aversion to intake, emaciation, normal general spirit, normal urine and stool, white or thin and greasy fur.

- Differentiation guidelines: normal spirit and physical activities, no appetite, emaciation, pale tongue, thin and whitish fur.

- Therapeutic principle: regulating stomach and harmonizing middle *jiao*, invigorating spleen to promote transportation.

- Treatment: clearing manipulation on stomach-meridian point, pushing spleen-meridian point to and fro, pushing four-transverse-crease point. (Picture 4–96 to Picture 4–98)

- Prescription analysis: Clearing manipulation on stomach-meridian point can promote digestion and resolve food stagnation; pushing spleen-meridian point to and fro can invigorate the spleen and replenish *qi* to strengthen its transportation and transformation; pushing four-transverse-crease point aims to increase appetite by smoothing *qi* flow and remove food stagnation.

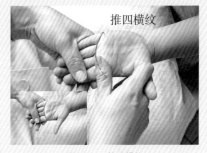

图 4-98　推四横纹
Picture 4–98　Pushing four-transverse-crease point

2　Deficiency of stomach *yin*

It is characterized as dry mouth, drinking favors, no appetite, dry and lusterless skin, dry and hard stool, red tongue, peeling fur and particularly red tongue.

- Differentiation guidelines: dry mouth, drinking favors, no appetite, peeling fur and particularly red tongue.

- Therapeutic principle: nourishing stomach *yin*.

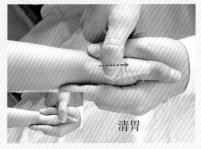

图 4-99　清胃
Picture 4–99　Clearing manipulation on stomach-meridian point

- Treatment: clearing manipulation on stomach-meridian point, pushing spleen-meridian point to and fro, kneading *erma* point. (Picture

135

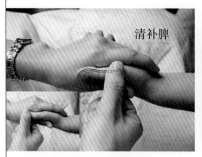

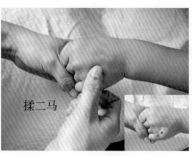

图 4-100 清补脾
Picture 4-100 Pushing spleen-meridian
point to and fro

图 4-101 揉二马
Picture 4-101 Kneading *erma* point

3. 脾胃气虚

精神较差，懒言，面色萎黄，厌食、拒食，若稍进饮食，大便中夹有不消化残渣，或大便不成形，容易出汗，舌淡苔薄。

辨证要点　精神较差，懒言，面色萎黄，多汗，拒食，舌淡苔薄。

治则　健脾益气。

取穴　平肝　清胃　清补脾（图 4-102～图 4-104）

方义　清肝经以疏肝和胃而助纳运；清胃经可开胃消食而化积；清补脾经可健脾益气而助运化。

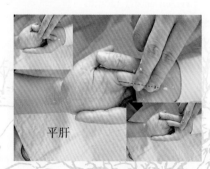

图 4-102 平肝
Picture 4-102 Clearing manipulation on liver-
meridian point

4 – 99 to Picture 4 – 101)

• Prescription analysis: Clearing manipulation on stomach-meridian point aims to promote digestion and resolve food stagnation; pushing spleen-meridian point to and fro can invigorate the spleen and replenish *qi* to strengthen its transportation and transformation; kneading *erma* point can aid in digestion by nourishing stomach *yin*.

3 *Qi*-deficiency of spleen and stomach

It is characterized as spiritless, reluctant to speak, sallow complexion, no appetite, or even aversion to food, undigested food dregs in stool even with a bit of eating, or loose stool, excessive sweating, pale tongue and thin fur.

• Differentiation guidelines: spiritless, reluctant to speak, sallow complexion, excessive sweating, no appetite, or even aversion to food, pale tongue, and thin fur.

• Therapeutic principle: invigorating spleen and replenishing *qi*.

• Treatment: clearing manipulation on liver-meridian point and stomach-meridian point, and pushing spleen-meridian point to and fro. (Picture 4 – 102 to Picture 4 – 104)

• Prescription analysis: Clearing manipulation on liver-meridian point aims to strengthen its transportation and transformation by soothing the liver and harmonizing the stomach; Clearing manipulation on stomach-meridian point aims to promote digestion and resolve food stagnation; pushing spleen-meridian point to and fro can invigorate the spleen and replenish *qi* to strengthen its transportation and transformation.

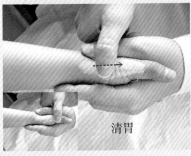

图 4 – 103 清胃
Picture 4 – 103 Clearing manipulation on stomach-meridian point

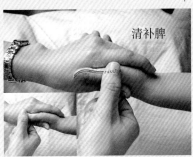

图 4 – 104 清补脾
Picture 4 – 104 Pushing spleen-meridian point to and fro

预防与护理

（1）**科普宣教是预防厌食症的有效方法** 小儿进食受家庭环境、情绪等因素影响很大，有时进食量会有波动，短期的食欲不振，生长发育、精神、活动各方面正常，不应视为厌食症。由于父母亲过分关爱孩子，认为把小儿喂养得越胖越好，当小儿的进食量达不到自己期望的标准或不如别人小孩胖时，就认为是厌食，实际上小儿摄入的食物已满足正常需要，生长发育在正常儿童标准范围内，这不属厌食，要让家长充分认识到这一点，科普宣教是有效的方法之一。

（2）**养成良好的饮食习惯是预防厌食症的有效措施** 现代家庭多为独生子女家庭，经济条件优越，对子女过度关爱而忽视了饮食卫生。诱骗、强迫进食造成小儿的逆反心理，不定时进食和吃零食过多破坏了消化系统的正常规律，这些不良的饮食习惯导致了小儿厌食；家庭不和睦，父母经常吵架、离异，小儿长期情绪紧张、抑郁、忧虑，这些精神因素也是导致小儿厌食的原因。养成良好的饮食习惯，保持愉快的就餐环境是防止小儿厌食的有效措施。

（3）**小儿厌食症的护理** 当小儿不进食时，千万不能露出急躁情绪，从小量进餐开始，逐渐增加；先从喜欢吃的开始，逐渐增加食物种类，限制吃零食，进餐不可过饱，留有余地，使其产生饥饿感，建立起正常的摄食习惯。避免体力过度劳累，精神过度紧张，而影响食欲和食量。

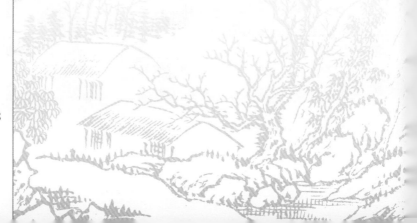

Prevention and Care

1 The popular science education is an effective way to prevent anorexia: Children's appetite is influenced by family environment, emotional and other factors greatly. Sometimes short-term loss of appetite with normal growth, development, vigor and activity should not be considered as anorexia. Nowadays parents love their baby too much, if the baby cannot eat as much as his/her parents expect, or the baby is not as fat as the others, which is mistaken for anorexia by their parents. Those children actually have eaten enough food to meet their normal needs, their growth and development is in the normal standard range, and therefore the condition does not pertain to anorexia. To let the parents fully aware of this, the popular science education is one of the effective ways.

2 It is an effective measure to prevent anorexia that develops a good eating habit: Now most family has one-child, its economic condition is superior, parents excessively care for their children, and ignore food hygiene. The children often have reverse psychology due to being tricked or forced to eat. Eating irregularly and snacking too much damage the normal rules of the digestive system leading to anorexia. Such psychological factors as family disharmony, frequent quarrelling and divorce of parents, prolonged emotional stress, depression, anxiety also cause anorexia. It is an effective measure to prevent anorexia that develop a good eating habit and keep a pleasant dining environment.

3 Care of children with anorexia: When children do not like eating, parents had better not show impatience, let children eat small amounts firstly and have more food gradually. Feed children with their favorite food, increase the kinds of food gradually, limit snacking, eating not too full, leaving room to produce a sense of hunger, and establish a normal feeding habit. Avoid excessive physical exertion, mental stress, which affect appetite and food intake.

第九节　夜啼

婴儿入夜啼哭不安，时哭时止，或每夜定时啼哭，甚至通宵达旦，但白天能安静入睡者称为夜啼。多见于新生儿及6个月以内的小婴儿。足够的睡眠是小儿健康的重要保证，啼哭不止，睡眠不足，生长发育就会受到影响。

病因病机

婴儿脏腑幼嫩，阴阳二气稚弱，调节能力差，环境适应能力低下，不论外感六淫还是内伤乳食，都可导致脏腑功能失调，阴阳气血失于平衡，只能用啼哭来表达痛苦。

脾寒腹痛是导致夜啼的常见原因。脾为太阴，为阴中之至阴，喜温而恶寒。若孕妇素体虚寒，恣食生冷，胎禀不足，脾寒乃生；或因调护失宜，腹部中寒，以致寒邪内侵，凝滞气机，不通则痛，因痛而啼。由于夜间属阴，阴胜则脾寒越盛，故啼在夜间。白天阳气盛，阴寒之气得阳而暂散，故白天能安然入睡。

若孕妇内蕴郁热，恣食辛热之食，或过服温热药物，蕴蓄之热遗于胎儿；或婴儿过温，受火热之气薰灼，心火上炎，心中懊恼，烦躁而啼。夜间阴盛阳衰，阳入于阴则入静而寐，由于心火过亢，阴不能潜阳，故夜间不寐而啼哭不止。彻夜啼哭后，阳气耗损，无力抗争，故白天入寐；正气未复，入夜又啼，周而复始，循环不已。

心主惊而藏神，小儿神气怯弱，若暴受惊恐，惊则伤神，恐则伤志，神志不宁，寐中惊惕，因惊而啼。

此外，不良习惯也可导致小儿夜啼，如夜间开灯而寐，摇篮中摇摆而寐，怀抱而寐，边走边抱而寐等。

Section 9   Night Crying

Night crying is a kind of disease in which infants are restless, cry on and off, in the evening, or cry at a certain time in the evening and even cry all through the night, while they are quiet and fall asleep in the day. It is much more common in infants less than 6 months. Sufficient sleep is essential to infantile health. If infants cry too much such that they do not have enough sleep, their growth and development will be affected.

Cause and mechanism of disease

Infantile viscera are tender and their constitutions are immature. Due to their weak ability of regulation and adaptation, they are vulnerable to external six excesses and internal injury of food, leading to disharmony of visceral function and imbalance of *qi*, blood, *yin*, and *yang*, through which they can only express by crying.

A common cause is abdominal pain of spleen cold. Spleen is *taiyin*, the extreme *yin* within *yin*, which is in favor of warm and detesting cold. If a deficiency- cold pregnant woman is partial to raw and cold foods, the fetus endowment will be insufficient and coldness in the fetus spleen will be engendered. When the infantile abdomen is invaded by cold-evil due to improper nursing, the cold-evil will go inward and clog *qi* movement. Cold accumulation and clogged *qi* movement result in stagnation. Stagnation leads to pain and infants cry due to the pain. The night belongs to *yin*, and when the *yin* prevails, the spleen cold flourishes. Contrary to the condition mentioned above, when *yang* prevails in the daytime, *yin* and cold are temporarily dispelled. So infants cry in the evening and fall asleep in the daytime.

Moreover, if a pregnant woman has internal heat accumulation and is particular to acrid and hot foods, or has too many warm and hot drugs, the accumulated heat will be transferred to fetus. If an infant is stricken by heat pathogen, heat burns internally and the heart fire flames upward. So the heart is upset and infants cry due to dysphoria. In the evening, *yin* prevails and *yang* declines. If *yang* submits to *yin*, people will be quiet and fall asleep. However, if heart fire is overwhelming, *yin* is unable to subdue *yang*, leading to insomnia and cry in the evening. Crying all night results

141

辨证施治

1. 脾虚中寒

入夜啼哭，时哭时止，哭声低弱，兼恶寒蜷卧，四肢不温，纳少便溏，肠鸣腹胀，口唇淡白，舌淡红苔薄白。

辨证要点　入夜啼哭，时哭时止，哭声低弱，纳少便溏，舌淡红苔薄白。

治则　温脾散寒，镇静安神。

取穴　补脾　揉外劳宫　捣小天心　掐五指节（图4-105～图4-108）

方义　补脾经可健脾益气以滋后天之本；揉外劳宫可温中散寒而缓解腹痛，使夜间安然入睡；捣小天心、掐五指节可镇惊安神而止啼。

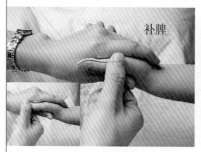

图4-105　补脾
Picture 4-105　Nourishing manipulation on spleen-meridian point

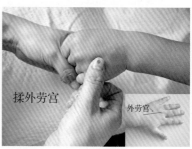

图4-106　揉外劳宫
Picture 4-106　Kneading dorsal-*laogong* point

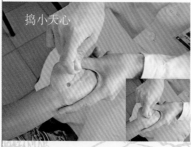

图4-107　捣小天心
Picture 4-107　Pounding small-heaven-center point

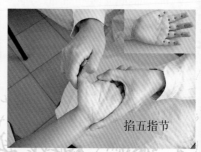

图4-108　掐五指节
Picture 4-108　Nipping finger-knuckle point

in the loss of *yang qi*, then, *yang* will submit to *yin* and there will be sleep in the daytime. Because healthy *qi* has not resumed, infants cry in the evening again. It is so that the night crying circles.

Heart governs fright and stores spirit. Infantile spirit is weak. If infants are stricken by panic in a sudden, fright will impair spirit, and fear will impair will. The result of a disturbed mind is infants are frightened in sleep and cry due to fright.

In addition, bad habits lead to night crying: sleep with lights on in the evening, sleep in a cradle by swinging, sleep in the arms, sleep by carrying and walking and so on.

Treatment according to syndrome differentiation

1 Cold stroke into deficient spleen

It is characterized as intermittent crying in the night, low voice, accompanied with aversion to cold, huddling, cool limbs, no appetite, loose stool, borborygmus, distension in abdomen, pale lips, pale red tongue, and thin and white fur.

* Differentiation guidelines: intermittent crying in the night, low voice, no appetite, loose stool, pale red tongue, and thin and white fur.

* Therapeutic principle: warming spleen to dispel cold, inducing sedation and tranquilization.

* Treatment: nourishing manipulation on spleen-meridian point, kneading dorsal-*laogong* point, pounding small-heaven-center point, and nipping finger-knuckle point. (Picture 4 – 105 to Picture 4 – 108)

* Prescription analysis: Nourishing manipulation on spleen-meridian point can nourish acquired root by invigorating the spleen and replenish *qi*; kneading dorsal-*laogong* point aims to relieve pain by warming the middle *jiao* and expelling cold; pounding small-heaven-center point and nipping finger-knuckle point can stop crying by calming fright and tranquilizing mind.

2. 心热内扰

入夜啼哭，哭声宏亮，见灯尤甚，烦躁不宁，面红唇赤，大便干结，小便浑浊，舌尖红，苔薄黄。

辨证要点　入夜啼哭，哭声宏亮，见灯尤甚，烦躁不宁，舌尖红。

治则　清心散热，镇静安神。

取穴　平肝　清胃　清天河水　捣小天心　掐五指节（图4-109～图4-113）

方义　平肝经以清肝泻火，镇惊除烦；清胃经以清中焦之热，消积除烦；清天河水以清心热而除心烦；捣小天心、掐五指节可镇惊安神而止啼。

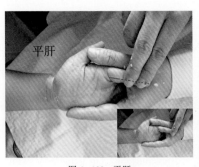

图4-109　平肝
Picture 4-109　Clearing manipulation on liver-meridian point

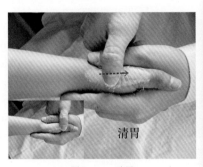

图4-110　清胃
Picture 4-110　Clearing manipulation on stomach-meridian point

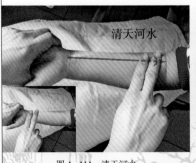

图4-111　清天河水
Picture 4-111　Clearing manipulation on heaven-river-water point

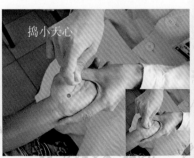

图4-112　捣小天心
Picture 4-112　Pounding small-heaven-center point

2　Internal disturbance of heart-heat

It is characterized as crying in the night, high voice, aggravated by seeing lights, dysphoria, restlessness, flushed complexion, red lips, dry and hard stool, turbid urination, red tongue tip, and thin and yellowish fur.

- Differentiation guidelines: crying in the night, high voice, aggravated by seeing lights, dysphoria, restlessness, and red tongue tip.

- Therapeutic principle: clearing heart-fire and dispelling heat, and inducing sedation and tranquilization.

- Treatment: clearing manipulation on liver-meridian point, stomach-meridian point and heaven-river-water point, pounding small-heaven-center point, and nipping finger-knuckle point. (Picture 4 – 109 to Picture 4 – 113)

- Prescription analysis: Clearing manipulation on liver-meridian point aims to clear the liver, purge fire, calm fright, and eliminate vexation; clearing manipulation on stomach-meridian point aims to clear heat in the middle *jiao*, remove food stagnation and eliminate vexation; clearing manipulation on heaven-river-water point aims to clear heart heat and eliminate vexation; pounding small-heaven-center point and nipping finger-knuckle point can stop crying by calming fright and tranquilizing mind.

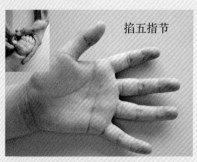

图 4 – 113　掐五指节
Picture 4 – 113　Nipping finger-knuckle point

3. 暴受惊恐

入夜而啼，啼声较尖，时作惊惕，紧偎母怀，面色乍青乍白，哭声时高时低，时急时缓，舌质正常。

辨证要点　入夜而啼，啼声较尖，时作惊惕，紧偎母怀，哭声时高时低。

治则　镇静安神。

取穴　平肝　清补脾　清天河水　捣小天心　掐五指节（图4-114～图118）

方义　平肝经以镇惊安神，平肝息风；与清天河水合用加强清心安神之功；清补脾经意在健脾益气而固后天之本；捣小天心、掐五指节可镇惊安神而止啼。

预防与护理

（1）小儿夜啼应当首先寻找原因，如饥饿、过饱、闷热、寒冷、虫咬、尿布浸湿、衣物刺激皮肤等，细心观察，去其原因，啼哭自止。

（2）孕妇、乳母应注意不过食寒凉及辛辣性食物，对婴幼儿要使其养成良好的睡眠习惯，不抱在怀中睡，不通宵开启灯具。

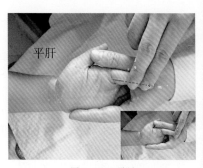

图4-114　平肝
Picture 4-114　Clearing manipulation on liver-meridian point

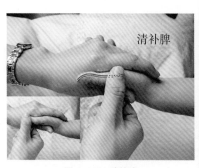

图4-115　清补脾
Picture 4-115　Pushing spleen-meridian point to and fro

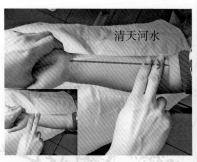

图4-116　清天河水
Picture 4-116　Clearing manipulation on heaven-river-water point

3 Panic stricken

It is characterized as harsh crying in the night, occasional frightened reactions, holding much more firmly, looming blue of pale complexion, fluctuating voice of crying, and normal tongue.

- Differentiation guidelines: harsh crying in the night, occasional frightened reactions, holding much more firmly, and fluctuating voice of crying.
- Therapeutic principle: inducing sedation and tranquilization.
- Treatment: clearing manipulation on liver-meridian point; pushing spleen-meridian point to and fro; clearing manipulation on heaven-river-water point, pounding small-heaven-center point, and nipping finger-knuckle point. (Picture 4 – 114 to Picture 4 – 118)
- Prescription analysis: Clearing manipulation on liver-meridian point aims to calm fright, tranquilize mind and calm liver wind; with heaven-river-water point, they can strengthen the function of clearing the heart and tranquilizing mind; pushing manipulation on spleen-meridian point to and fro aims to consolidate the acquired root by invigorating the spleen and replenishing qi; pounding small-heaven-center point and nipping finger-knuckle point can stop crying by calming fright and tranquilizing mind.

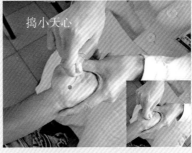

图 4 – 117 捣小天心
Picture 4 – 117   Pounding small-heaven-center point

Prevention and Care

1 Look for the causes first, such as hunger, fullness, hot, cold, insect bites, wet diapers, and other skin irritation caused by clothing. Observe carefully, give symptomatic treatment, and then the crying will stop.

2 Pregnant women and nursing mothers should not eat cold and spicy foods too much. Help infants develop a good sleep habit, do not let baby sleep either in mother's arms, or with light on all night.

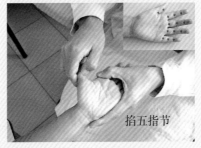

图 4 – 118   拍五指节
Picture 4 – 118   Nipping finger-knuckle point

147

第十节 奶麻

奶麻即幼儿急疹，是婴幼儿时期的一种病毒性出疹性疾病。临床特征为突然发热，持续高热3～4日后，热退出疹，疹点为红色粟粒状小红疹，散布全身，并很快消退。本病属中医温病范畴，由于出疹形态与麻疹相似，又好发于哺乳期小儿，因此，中医古代文献又将之称为"奶麻"。

病因病机

中医学认为，本病为外感风热时邪所致。风热时邪由口鼻而入，首伤肺卫，故初期见有肺卫表证，但为时短暂，继而邪郁化热，邪热蕴郁肺胃，肺胃气分热盛，故见高热，烦渴，或伴呕吐、泄泻、纳减等症。由于机体抗邪有力，热蕴肺胃数日，与气血相搏而发于肌肤，邪热得以外泄，故热退疹出。

辨证施治

1. 热蕴肺胃（发热期）

突然高热，常伴有咳嗽目赤，纳呆呕吐，或有烦躁，惊惕，咽微红肿，小便黄，舌偏红，苔薄黄。

辨证要点　突然高热，常伴有目赤，咽微红肿，小便黄，舌偏红，苔薄黄。

治则　疏风清热。

取穴　平肝清肺　清胃退六腑（图4-119～图4-121）

方义　平肝经可行气解郁，以防肝火旺盛；清肺经有疏风解表而透疹的作用；清胃经有清热泻火的作用；退六腑有通腑泄热的作用。

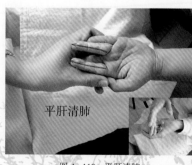

平肝清肺

图4-119　平肝清肺
Picture 4-119　Clearing manipulation on liver-meridian point and lung-meridian point

Section 10　Roseola Infantum

Roseola infantum, namely infantile acute rash, is a kind of rash infected by virus in the stage of an infant. It is characterized as abrupt onset of fever, continuous high fever for about 3 to 4 days, with occurrence of rash after recovery from fever. The form of rash is similar to that of measles, which is a kind of red granule. The red granules spread all over the body and disappear soon after. Roseola infantum belongs to warm disease in TCM.

Cause and mechanism of disease

In TCM, this disease is caused by external contraction wind-heat of epidemic pathogen. When wind-heat of epidemic pathogen strikes through mouth and nose, it impairs lung and defense phase at first. So, in early stage, there will be the defensive exterior syndrome of lung. After a short period, the stagnated pathogen generates heat, which accumulates in lung and stomach, leading to exuberant heat in *qi* phase of lung and stomach. As a result, it manifests as high fever, vexing, thirsty, or accompanied with vomiting, diarrhea, losing appetite, and so on. After days of heat accumulation in lung and stomach, if the body is strong enough to repel the pathogen, the heat will combat with *qi* and blood, then be dispelled outwards, which has the manifestation on skin. Resultantly, the heat goes down and rash comes out.

Treatment according to syndrome differentiation

1　Heat accumulation in lung and stomach (fever stage)

It is characterized by abrupt onset of high fever, often accompanied with cough, red eyes, anorexia, vomiting, or dysphoria, frightened reaction, slightly flared throat, yellow urine, particularly red tongue, and thin and yellow fur.

- Differentiation guidelines: abrupt onset of high fever, often accompanied with red eyes, slightly flared throat, yellow urine, particularly red tongue, and thin and yellow fur.
- Therapeutic principle: dispelling wind and clearing heat.
- Treatment: clearing manipulation on liver-meridian point, lung-meridian point, stomach-meridian point, and six-*fu* point. (Picture 4－119

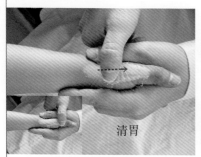

清胃

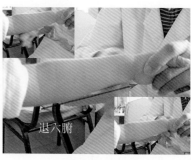

退六腑

图 4-120 清胃
Picture 4-120 Clearing manipulation on
stomach-meridian point

图 4-121 退六腑
Picture 4-121 Clearing manipulation on six-*fu*
point

2. 热透肌肤（出疹期）

热退，全身皮肤出现玫瑰色小丘疹，可融合成片，无痒感，出疹 2～3 日消退，舌偏红，苔黄。

辨证要点　热退，全身皮肤出现玫瑰色小丘疹，无痒感，舌偏红，苔黄。

治则　养阴清热。

取穴　平肝清肺　清天河水　揉二马（图 4-122～图 4-124）

方义　平肝经疏肝解郁；清肺经宣肺透表；清天河水具有清热泻火而不伤阴的作用；揉二马具有养阴清热而退余热的作用。

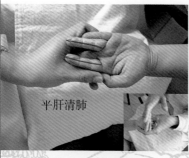

平肝清肺

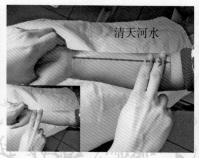

清天河水

图 4-122 平肝清肺
Picture 4-122 Clearing manipulation on
liver-meridian point and lung-meridian point

图 4-123 清天河水
Picture 4-123 Clearing manipulation on heaven-
river-water point

to Picture 4 – 121)

• Prescription analysis: Clearing manipulation on liver-meridian point can promote *qi* flow and relieve depression to avoid excessive liver fire; clearing manipulation on lung-meridian point can promote eruption by expelling wind and relieving exterior syndrome; clearing manipulation on stomach-meridian point can clear heat and purge fire; clearing manipulation on six-*fu* point can purge *fu*-organs to eliminate heat.

2   Heat penetration through skin (rash stage)

It is characterized by recovery from fever, rosy spots of papule all over the body, sometimes stuck in pieces, not itchy, rash disappearing in 2 to 3 days, particular red tongue, and yellow fur.

• Differentiation guidelines: recovery from fever, rosy spots of papule all over the body, not itchy, particularly red tongue, and yellow fur.

• Therapeutic principle: nourishing *yin* and clearing heat.

• Treatment: clearing manipulation on liver-meridian point, lung-meridian point and heaven-river-water point, and kneading *erma* point. (Picture 4 – 122 to Picture 4 – 124)

• Prescription analysis: Clearing manipulation on liver-meridian point aims to soothe the liver and relieve depression; clearing manipulation on lung-meridian point aims to ventilate the lung to relieve exterior syndrome; clearing manipulation on heaven-river-water point can clear heat, purge fire without damaging *yin*; kneading *erma* point can nourish *yin* and clear heat to clear residual heat.

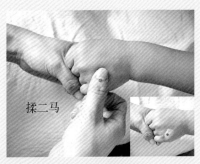

图 4 – 124   揉二马
Picture 4 – 124   Kneading *erma* point

预防与护理

（1）对高热患儿要及时对症处理，防止高热惊厥。

（2）多饮白开水，避免风寒，以防汗出当风。

（3）饮食宜清淡易消化。

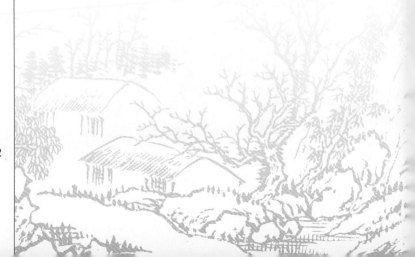

Prevention and Care

1 Give children with high fever symptomatic treatment promptly to prevent febrile convulsion.

2 Drink enough boiled water, avoid wind and cold, and prevent sweating in the wind.

3 Feed children with a light and digestible diet.

编　后　语

　　小儿推拿是医生用于治疗的一种方法，小儿推拿的成败在于疗效，而疗效之关键在于人，因此，可以说小儿推拿成败的关键也在于人。对推拿医生手法最基本的要求是持久、有力、均匀、柔和，从而达到"深透"的目的。

　　怎样才能达到基本要求：掌握推拿知识是基础，锻炼手法能力是关键，热爱推拿工作是核心，三者相互关联，形成稳定的三维结构，完善的三维结构是成为高素质推拿师的必备条件，也是不断消除影响小儿推拿临床疗效不利因素的必备条件。

　　任何一种治疗都有其局限性，小儿推拿更是如此。小儿推拿疗法并不是以消除原始致病因素及逆转病理变化为特长，而是从总体上对小儿的各种功能状态进行整体性调节。在临床诊治中如何针对小儿病症进行综合分析，选择最佳的切入点，是小儿推拿临床工作的要点。试举案例说明如下。

　　案例一　王某，男，7个月。主诉：鼻塞、咳嗽2日。患儿2日前因家人感冒而后出现鼻塞、咳嗽，体温正常，食欲减退，未用药物。查体：一般情况良好，咽部充血，舌苔白厚，心肺听诊无异常。系外感咳嗽，予以疏风解表、宣肺止咳，取穴：运八卦5分钟，平肝清肺10分钟，清胃10分钟。次日复诊，鼻塞消失，偶咳，查体咽部充血明显减轻，重复上方，嘱无需复诊。

案例二　秦某，男，5个月。发热、咳嗽10日。患儿7日前因发热、咳嗽3日在外院确诊为支气管肺炎，静滴7日，仍发热、咳嗽，喉中痰声辘辘，食欲差，3日未排便，要求中医治疗。查体：一般情况良好，体温37.8℃，两肺布满痰鸣音，舌苔白腻。系内伤咳嗽（痰湿阻肺证），予以通腑泄热，宣肺止咳，取穴：退六腑10分钟，平肝清肺10分钟，清补脾10分钟，嘱家长停用所有药物，多饮水。翌日复诊，当晚体温正常，咳嗽减轻，清晨排便1次，喉中痰鸣消失，两肺呼吸音粗，闻及少许痰鸣音，予以清肺10分钟，清补脾10分钟，运八卦5分钟，连续治疗2日而愈。

小儿推拿是医生根据病情，以不同的、轻柔的推拿手法作用于人体体表的特定部位从而调节机体的生理病理状况，达到治疗和保健的目的。小儿推拿手法是良性的、有序的和具有双向调节性的物理刺激，易被小儿内脏或形体感知，从而产生功效。临床实际操作中，医生正确的判断，恰当的选择，是十分重要的。案例一是外感咳嗽的初期，顺运八卦能宽胸顺气而化痰；清肝经行气化痰而止咳；清肺经解表宣肺，化痰止咳；清胃经意在利咽止咳。案例二是痰湿阻肺证，肺与大肠相表里，腑气不通，肺气何降，退六腑清热通腑以除痰浊，腑气通而咳骤减，继而调理则愈。

小儿推拿的生存与发展，需要一个良好的社会氛围，这不仅需要人们对小儿推拿的认识不断加深，同时需要小儿推拿的品牌建设。技术品牌和服务品牌是小儿推拿生存与发展的载体。作为技术品牌，应当着眼于国际医疗市场，在这方面我们有强大的优势，如何发挥这一优势，还需要一定的政策扶持；作为服务品牌，是医疗单位综合素质的体现，其本身就是诚信，是来自以质量为本的经营努力。

小儿推拿蕴含了有益于人类自身健康发展的新理念，也是 21 世纪的热门学科。

Additional Words

Pediatric massage is a kind of therapeutic method, the curative effect of massage depends on the clinical procedures of the doctor. The basic requirement for the manipulation should be permanent, forceful, even and soft so as to be deep and thorough.

How to do pediatric massage well? The basis rests with grasping the knowledge of massage; the key lies with strict training of manipulation; and the core is the love for massage. The three points are interrelated and form a stable three-dimensional structure which is prerequisite for becoming a high-quality massager as well as eliminating the unfavorable factors influencing the curative effect of pediatric massage.

Any kind of therapeutic method has its limit, so does the pediatric massage. The superiority of the pediatric massage does not lie with eliminating original pathogenic factors and the reversing the pathological changes, but with a whole regulation of the children on various functional states. How to comprehensively analyze infantile diseases and select the best starting point in clinical diagnosis and treatment is the key point of the clinical work of pediatric massage. Just list two cases as follows.

Case 1. Wang, baby boy, 7 months. Chief complaint: stuffy nose and cough for 2 days. The baby became stuffy and had a cough caused by his family member with cold 2 days ago. He manifested as normal temperature, loss of appetite, no intake of drugs. PE: a good general condition, ingestion of the pharynx, thick white tongue fur, and normal

157

heart and lung auscultation. It was diagnosed as exogenous cough, therapy of it was repelling wind to release the exterior and ventilating the lung to relieve cough. Treatment: arc-pushing *bagua* point for 5 min, clearing liver-meridian point and lung-meridian point for 10 min, clearing stomach-meridian point for 10 min. The next day, the baby was not stuffy and had a little cough, pharyngeal hyperaemia was improved significantly. Continue the same therapy this time and then tell the baby's parents that the baby will not need a return visit.

Case 2. Qin, baby boy, 5 months. Chief complaint: fever and cough for 10 days. Because of three days of fever and cough, the baby was diagnosed bronchial pneumonia in other hospital 7 days ago. After 7 days of intravenous drip, he still had fever and cough with the sound of phlegm in the throat, poor appetite, no defecation for 3 days. PE: a good general condition, body temperature of 37.8°C, both lungs with a lot of phlegm sound, thick white tongue fur. It was endogenous cough with syndrome of phlegm-dampness accumulated in the lung, therapy of it was purging *fu*-organs to eliminate heat, ventilating the lung to relieve cough. Treatment: clearing six-*fu* point for 10 min, clearing liver-meridian point and lung-meridian point for 10 min, pushing spleen-meridian point to and fro for 10 min. Let the baby drink more water without taking drugs. Return visit in the next day: The baby had a normal body temperature and alleviated cough that night and manifested as defecation one time in the early morning, no phlegm sound in the throat, rough breath sound in both lungs with a little phlegm sound. Treatment: clearing lung-meridian point for 10 min, pushing spleen-meridian point to and fro for 10 min, arc-pushing *bagua* point for 5 min. The baby recovered after 2 days of therapy.

How does the pediatric massage work? Actually, to achieve treatment and healthcare aims, a manipulator applies different and gentle *tuina* (massage) manipulations to the specific points on the surface of human body to adjust the physiological and pathological conditions of organism according to child's condition. The pediatric massage manipulation is a sort of healthy, orderly physical stimulation with bidirectional adjusting effect, and is easily perceptible by internal organs or body of children and therefore it works. It is very important for a doctor to judge correctly and select therapy properly in clinical practice. In case 1, the baby was diagnosed with exogenous cough in the early stage. Arc-pushing *bagua* point clockwise was applied to resolve phlegm by freeing the chest and promoting *qi* flow; clearing liver-meridian point was used to relieve cough by promoting *qi* flow and eliminating phlegm; clearing lung-meridian point was used to release the exterior and ventilate the lung, and resolve phlegm and stop cough; clearing stomach-meridian point was used to relieve cough by relaxing the throat. In case 2, the baby was diagnosed with endogenous cough with syndrome of phlegm-dampness accumulated in the lung. Because the lung and the large intestine are interior-exteriorly related, lung-*qi* cannot descend if bowel-*qi* is obstructed. Clearing six-*fu* point was used to eliminate phlegm turbidity by purging *fu*-organs to eliminate heat and therefore cough was relieved quickly and recovered by recuperation.

Survival and development of the pediatric massage needs a good social atmosphere. People's better understanding and the brand construction of the pediatric massage are essential. Technology and service brands act as the carrier of survival and development of the pediatric massage. As a technology brand, the pediatric massage should focus on its international medical market and we have a strong advantage in this respect. How to develop the advantage? We need some policy support. As a service brand, it reflects the comprehensive quality of medical units, it is actually honesty, and is derived from quality-oriented efforts.

Pediatric massage contains some new ideas benefiting the health development of human beings and is also a hot subject in the 21st century.